Teaching and Evaluating the Affective Domain in Nursing Programs

Editor

Dorothy E. Reilly, R.N., Ed.D., F.A.A.N.

Professor of Nursing
College of Nursing
Wayne State University
Detroit, Michigan

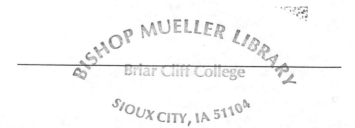

FIRST PRINTING — JUNE 1978
SECOND PRINTING — MARCH 1979
THIRD PRINTING — JUNE 1982

Preface

A Moment That Cried Out for Compassion

Despite my deep and crushing pain, I feel a dire need to share a tragic and dehumanizing, absolutely shattering experience.

Our daughter was taken to a hospital following an automobile accident of August 6. She had left home only a few hours earlier to spend the evening with friends. The next moment she was dead. Our big-little girl had been taken to a hospital's emergency room. We were called there. Doctors were on duty and in charge. Theirs was the voice that pronounced our Lore's end. We had every right to expect awareness of our overwhelming grief, tenderness toward our massive loss, calm to assist us through those first moments of shock.

Instead the doctor greeted us with, "Your daughter didn't make it." He insisted on immediate identification and immediate signature on the autopsy report, He insisted we wait for the police. And the nurse said, "Don't worry about it. We see this every day."

Whether by instinct, character or training, these "helpers" hurt two distraught parents. We needed human help. They insisted on bureaucratic protocol. We needed a moment to hold our hearts. They insisted on immediate action. We needed to retreat to our home to grasp our grief. They insisted we await the uniformed authorities.

Months have passed since then. We are learning to deal with our agonies and grief, but those words continue to ring in my ears and haunt my very silence. We were bowed in dismayed grief. Impersonal pronouncements perhaps protected doctoral pain. They added considerably to ours.

Doctors, please search yourselves for resources to deal helpfully with others like us. Seek ways to make the few moments available for deeply troubled persons times of healing rather than destruction. Plan ways of staffing your facilities with, or have immediately available to them, someone who is full of heart and wise in the administration of compassion. We need caring, so desperately.

Lore Kruger*

Potomac

*Kruger L: Letter to the editor. Washington Post. 3 March 1977.

On March 3, 1977, Lore Kruger used the column of the *Washington Post* Letter to the Editor to address health care providers. Her plea is for humanistic caring. She asks us to transcend our procedures, routines, and our veneer acquired through constant exposure to tragedy to see the persons who are seeking our care. In essence, we must reach out to our fellow beings and protect the integrity of the human being wherever we encounter him. Lore reminds us of the tremendous vulnerability of those who come to us in tragedy.

Lore Kruger is speaking to us as nurses. We belong to a profession whose essence and reason for being is the assistance of individuals in matters of health. Our code of ethics and our standards for practice recognize the totality of man's nature and charge us to be prepared to assist an individual as he responds to all dimensions of living such as joy, sorrow, fear, hope, and pain. Our methodology, nursing process, provides us with a framework for individualizing our care so that the integrity of the client can be protected at all times.

However, in most of our educational programs, do we teach to our practitioners the skills essential for working with the concept of man's totality? Competency in cognitive and psychomotor skills is generally identified as a goal of most educational programs within nursing schools and staff development programs in health care agencies. They are taught within these programs subject to disciplined pedagogy. What about skills in the affective domain? These skills are acknowledged as essential to nursing ministrations, but unfortunately they are not subjected to the same rigorous pedagogy as are the other domains.

Skills in interpersonal relationships are sought for all learners as nursing recognizes its human transactional nature heavily dependent upon communication competency in its practitioners. The process is taught as a skill to be integrated with all the other skills inherent in nursing practice.

What happens, however, with the interface of the care giver and the care receiver? The field of each intersects as the transaction becomes operational. Each person's field carries with it the needs, values, beliefs, interests, and aspirations of the participant. Nursing assessment skills, essential for planning patient care, incorporate the gathering of data about these affective components of the client's field.

But what about the field of the giver? What affective components does the giver bring to the transaction and how do these components influence the interpretation of the client's field? Are there certain affective components that are a critical part of any nurse's field and need to be developed during the educational program? If the response is affirmative, then the development of affective competencies must be subjected to the same pedagogy as other nursing competencies.

Several faculty members of the College of Nursing at Wayne State University believe that the affective component of nursing care can be taught with the same disciplined approach used for the other domains of learning. They developed a workshop, "Teaching and Evaluating the Affective Domain in Nursing Programs," addressed to these critical issues of ethical, moral, and value development. The intent is to introduce (or reintroduce) nursing faculty to current theories which they may use in developing the affective component of their curriculum. The papers presented and the moral and value exercises used at the various workshops are incorporated in the monograph.

Ann Zuzich describes some of the ethical frameworks which are or may be used by individuals in making ethical decisions. Identifying the roots in Greek philosophy, Zuzich presents concepts of Christian ethics, Judaic ethics, situation ethics, and structural ethics. She concludes by relating the need for examining more closely the interplay between the ethical domain and the technological progress we are making through our scientific inquiry process.

Mary Castles examines the incongruences between our stated professional code and our personal values. Castles describes the two value systems and their impact on the choices that nurses have in making professional decisions relative to the care of clients. She presents issues where the professional code may not reflect personal values or where current accepted practices are not congruent with the professional code.

Darimell Waugh presents Kohlberg's Theory of Moral Development as a useful framework for teaching the moral component in a nursing program. Each of the developmental stages are examined and related to nursing practice behaviors. Waugh illustrates the various behaviors characteristic of each stage through a cheating incident involving two nursing students.

Dorothy Reilly states that values can be taught and describes the valuing process as conceptualized by Raths and the relationship of that process to the taxonomy of the affective domain as developed by Krathwohl, et al. Strategies for teaching values, which emphasize experiencing and critical thinking, are currently being used in most programs. Reilly urges that the present strategies be enlarged to encompass the affective component.

Dorothy Reilly follows her thesis that the affective domain can be taught by demonstrating that it can also be subjected to a rigorous evaluation protocol as is developed for the other two domains, cognitive and psychomotor. Emphasizing climate appropriate for affective evaluation, evaluation strategies relative to experiencing and critical thinking are presented. A taxonomy of behaviors and evaluation strategies for implementing one of the nursing standards is presented.

Ann Zuzich presents a summary that was given at each workshop following the activities which included the presentation of papers and group process relative to moral and value decisions in nursing.

The *Appendix* includes the moral decision group activities and the value decision group activities which were presented at the workshop.

The authors of this monograph wish to extend special appreciation to the participants who attended the workshops sponsored by the College of Nursing/College of Lifelong Learning, Wayne State University in Detroit, Michigan; George Mason University in Fairfax, Virginia; Fanshawe College in London, Ontario; and Iowa Lakes Community College in Emmetsburg, Iowa.

The enthusiasm and involvement of the participants contributed greatly to the growth of the presenters and supported their efforts to produce this monograph.

Dorothy E. Reilly, R.N., Ed.D., F.A.A.N.
Professor of Nursing
Wayne State University

July 31, 1977

Table of Contents

1

Some Frameworks for Ethical Development

Ann Zuzich, R.N., M.S.

The values that we hold are reflected in the behavior that we demonstrate. That behavior has been the focus of study of great thinkers since Socrates, who is usually considered to have begun the discipline of ethical thought.

A generally accepted definition of ethics is the study of standards of conduct and moral judgment. Greek philosophy considered what is ultimately good or desirable for man as the primary subject of ethical investigation. Stent offers a more sophisticated definition, the development of which he attributes to J. M. Gustafson: "Ethics is a human intellectual discipline which develops the principles which account for morality and moral action and the normative principles and values that are to guide human action."[1]

Traditional Ethical Concepts

The continuing evolvement of ethical thought since Socrates has provided a variety of frameworks within which principles have been proposed to account for moral action. It is hoped that this very brief presentation of some of the concepts from those frameworks will provide some bases for thought about your own ethical development.

What are the normative principles and values that guide human action?

What is "ultimately good and desirable for man"?

Since the early Greeks, the identification of "the good" has been a consistent problem for philosophers. The Hedonistic school defined the good as pleasure. G. E. Moore, opposed to all forms of Hedonistic utilitarianism, concluded that the "good" is simple, not analyzable, and indefinable, and at the same time proceeded to develop his utilitarianism

Ann Zuzich

framework on the concept of "good," intuitively known as a most
important term. Moore recognized pleasure as a necessary component of
things that are good, but he did not believe that good means pleasure.

Christian ethics proposed that the origin of the "good" is the Maker of
all things and the Light by which all things are known. It is based upon
divine revelation which demands an act of faith. The human being, as a
creature of God, yearns for reunion with the creator who is all truth and
all goodness. Progress toward that reunion is only possible through the
gifts of divine grace of knowledge and love. St. Paul explains the meaning
of love:

> Love is patient; love is kind. Love is not jealous, it does not put on airs, it is not
> snobbish. Love is never rude, it is not self-seeking, it is not prone to anger, neither
> does it brood over injuries. Love does not rejoice in what is wrong but rejoices with
> the truth. There is no limit to love's forebearance, to its trust, its hope, its power to
> endure.[2]

Christian love or "agape" is usually distinguished from friendship love
(phylia) and romantic love (eros). The object of agape is "neighbor" —
meaning everybody. It is a love effected through the will and it motivates
Christian behavior. It is a central focus of Christian ethics.

Banner interprets St. Augustine,

> To know and to reach God as the chief good is to accept the divine order concerning
> oneself and one's neighbor. To love what is best for oneself is to love oneself and to
> love others as individuals capable of likeness to God. To obey the precepts of love is
> to support the aspirations of all men to live well and happily. From this precept
> proceed all the duties of human society.[3]

To fulfill the yearning for reunion with the creator while accepting the
divine order concerning oneself and one's neighbor necessitates the
assistance of divine grace. Fundamental is the act of faith.

The concept of duty is the basis for legalistic morality. The Judaic
tradition expresses such a legalistic framework. It is historically the
precedent for the development of Christian morality. The ancient Jews
lived by the law or *Torah*. Laws necessarily multiplied in order to apply to
every conceivable situation. Following the letter of the law became very
restrictive. Reformed Jews, straining under those restrictions, have
become released from the formal adherence to the law that is still the
basis of orthodoxy.

Catholic Christian ethics also embody the concept of the natural law
which is the "Divine Will or the Divine Order as grasped by human
reason and as setting forth principles of individual and social morality

which are binding upon all men."[3] It is in the study of nature that God's will can be discerned. To act unnaturally is to defy God's will and to depart from that pursuit which leads to the finding of God.

In our day the concept of the natural law has generally fallen into disrepute. However, it is worthy of mention here because of its long tradition in Catholic Christian ethics as a viable theory. Jonsen proposes that it can still serve a very vital purpose if the concept can be considered as the statement of the basis for moral thought. He sees it as the determination of the basic potentialities and needs of the human person. Those characteristics of the human person which are the same at every time in every place are elucidated by the natural law. He suggests four of these: 1) man is capable of reflecting on himself and his actions; 2) man is capable of freely engaging himself in action that he chooses; 3) man is a being situated in history and he has a history and; 4) man develops as a person in interaction with other persons.[4] Man's behavior then is moral when these characteristics are protected and promoted.

According to the classical Christian ethicist, then, the "good" is God. Man knows what he ought to do through an act of faith, and he is assisted by the gifts of divine grace. He understands himself as a creature of God with an obligation to all other human beings in the promotion of their movement toward reunion with the Creator.

Situation Ethics

Fletcher describes Situation Ethics, or the New Morality, as in between legalism (laws for everything) and antinomianism or the lawless and unprincipled approach.

> The Situationist enters into every decision making situation fully armed with the ethical maxims of his community and its heritage, and he treats them with respect as illuminations of his problems. Just the same he is prepared in any situation to compromise them or set them aside in the situation if love seems better served by doing so.[5]

Six basic propositions explain the Situationist position:

Love alone is always good. The intrinsic "good" is love — "agape." Nothing is good in and of itself. It is good only if it helps persons. It is bad if it hurts persons.

The only ruling norm of Christian decision is love. Legalistic norms are rejected; the objectivity provided by the law is disputed. Moral decision making by the free man is always risky; the use of the law which may curtail creativity and responsibility diminishes the person. Decisions made within the ruling norm of Christian love and using all available facts are growth-producing and ethically sound.

Love and justice are the same. Fletcher sees that the thing that we owe our neighbor — the due — is only love, and he reasons that love is justice and justice is love. "Justice is Christian love using its head, calculating its duties, obligations, opportunities, resources.....justice is love coping with situations where distribution is called for. On this basis it becomes plain that as the love searches seriously for a social policy, it must form a coalition with utilitarianism."

Love is not liking. Love wills the neighbor's good whether we like him or not. Love is not emotional. It is volitional.

Only the end justifies the means — nothing else. The only way to justify any act is in a loving purpose. Evil means do not always nullify good ends; it depends upon the situation.

Love's decisions are made situationally, not prescriptively.

> The Situationist, cutting himself loose from the dead hand of unyielding law with its false promises of relief from the anguish of decision, can only determine that as a man of good will he will live as a free man, with all the ambiguities that go along with freedom. His moral life takes on the shape of adventure, ceases to pretend to be a blueprint. In all humility, knowing that he cannot escape the human margin of error, he will, in Luther's apposite phrase, "sin bravely."[5]

Situation Ethics then is a one-norm ethic. A single universal norm must be very broad in order for it to have applicability in all circumstances. And it is that necessary versatility that provokes doubt. What is meant by love? Fletcher says "love is not a substance...it is a principle, a formal principle, expressing what type of actions Christians are to call good." Fletcher seems to be saying that love as a universal norm has no concrete content outside of the relative situation. The meaning of love is dependent upon the circumstances.

In Situation Ethics, Fletcher uses many examples to explain the situationist position. Illustrating the proposition that love and justice are the same, he tells the story of the emergency room physician faced with the care of two critically injured patients — a young mother of three, and a skid-row drunk. He must decide which patient should receive the hospital's last unit of blood. Fletcher justifies the use of the blood for the young mother by saying that the most loving decision is to serve more rather than fewer — that is the just decision in the situationist's view. And again, he relates the story of the ship that struck an iceberg and sank. One of the boats that got away was loaded with seven seaman and thirty-two passengers — more than twice what it could hold. A seaman, acting on the mate's orders, ordered most of the male survivors into the sea and thus to their deaths. The rest of the party were eventually rescued. Later, on shore, the seaman was convicted of murder with mercy recommended. Fletcher believes that the seaman did not do an evil thing, but a good thing. He did, in fact, act "bravely sinful."

According to the Situationist, the "good" depends upon the situation. A loving purpose must underlie every moral act, but the act itself can only be evaluated ethically, contingent upon the circumstances surrounding its performance. The very lack of guidelines for the decision about the morality of any act places the responsibility for the decision solely on the shoulders of the actor. He alone determines the "good."

Structuralist Ethics
A Proposed Response to Legalism and/or Arbitrariness

Gunther Stent proposes a structuralist ethics. The possibility arises that there is an innate knowledge not derived from direct experience. The determinants of behavior, in this view, lie in this deep innate structure and are inaccessible to direct observation. And Stent suggests that the discovery of this deep structure ought to be the real goal of the human sciences.

To elucidate, Stent uses the concept of structuralism inherent in Chomsky's approach to linguistics.[6] Chomsky proposes that the surface structure of speech — or the sentence structure — is generated by the speaker from a covert deep structure. He believes that all men possess an innate knowledge of a universal grammar and, in spite of superficial differences, all languages are based on that grammar. The phonological component of language reflects the surface structure; the semantics component reflects the deep structure; and the syntactic component pairs the deep and surface structures. Some progress has been made in studying the surface structure of language, and some universal "distinctive features" have been identified. Less progress has been achieved in the study of the deep structure — universal semantic "distinctive features." However, the knowledge of the constancy through time of universal aspects of the deep structures and the surface structures has led to the belief that these can be attributed only to an innate, hereditary aspect of the mind. The study of structuralist linguistics continues in its pursuit of these universal aspects of grammar.

Structural ethics, in a similar way, holds that explanations of behavior must be formulated in terms of deep structures and transformational procedures. "Moral judgments arise by a generative process involving transformational operations on a subconscious mental deep structure."[1] Observations of the multitude of value judgments that can be made by man that will be acceptable to other men point to the idiosyncratic aspects of values. However, since all human beings share an ethical, universal deep structure, complete arbitrariness is avoided. The overt surface structure is the moral code of which the individual is aware, and which he can verbally express. The covert deep structure is the abstract moral code of which the individual is unaware and which he cannot express. This deep structure is innate and common to all men. Consistent with psychological thought, the primary course of the transformational process would be the assimilation of parental moral authority by the child. This is possible because the child already knows, thanks to the innate ethical deep structure, the meaning of concepts of moral values, such as "good."

Stent admits the difficulty in defining the moral content of the deep ethical structure. He suggests that Kant thought he had clearly defined it in his categorical imperative, namely, "Act only according to that maxim which you can will to be universal law." Kant did not, however, propose the surface structure concept along with the transformational process which Stent suggests as a framework for the creative aspect of morality.

Stent's background as a biologist is clearly evident. His understanding of the transformations that occur in the physiological processes that transform light rays on the retina of the eye into a visual perception is an example that he uses to explain the transformation phenomena in the ethical domain. Such a theory permits the individual creativity that is prohibited by legalistic frameworks and, at the same time, provides the universal norm within the deep mental structure. It is the potential for creativity that Stent believes provides the moral dilemmas that continually confront us; and he further suggests that there is no possibility for relief from these dilemmas short of redesigning the human being.

Some Frameworks for Ethical Development

The Relationship Between
Science and Ethics

The state of affairs in which currently we find ourselves in our highly technological society is stimulating the ethicists and moralists to evaluate our human progress. Contemporary scientific successes seem to far outdistance ethical successes. The sophistication of the scientific method of inquiry seems to exclude any application in the ethical domain. The view that science is "value-full" and that it is possible for men to pursue the ends of scientific inquiry unencumbered by ethical issues, is being seriously questioned. Modern philosophers are beginning to study the relationships between ethics and science to determine whether they are, in fact, mutually exclusive. A research group at the Institute of Society, Ethics, and the Life Sciences has been studying "The Foundations of Ethics and Its Relationships to the Sciences." At the end of their first year they have presented some interesting conclusions:

1. The images and metaphors of ethics are often borrowed from, and influenced by, theories of science and knowledge.

2. The sciences are structured by value judgments concerning what humans should be like and should be able to do.

3. Science and ethics, though conceptually indistinguishable, are, in fact, inseparable due to a web of interdependent concepts and ideas.

4. It is necessary to place the activities of science within the broader scope of human activities in general.

5. Ethics must be attentive to the knowledge of the empirical sciences.[7]

It is anticipated that additional light will be shed on the nature of the interplay between ethics and scientific inquiry.

Scientific progress has presented us with knowledge that has potential for our destruction. Identification of the ethical domain in the development of that scientific knowledge will permit humanistic concepts to have impact on the development of man.

References

1. Stent GS: The poverty of scientism and the promise of structuralist ethics. Hastings Center Report 6:39, December 1976.
2. 1 Corinthians 13:4-7.
3. Banner W: Ethics: An Introduction to Moral Philosophy. New York, Charles Scribner's Sons, 1968, pp 67, 73-74.
4. Jonsen AR: Christian Decision and Action. New York, Bruce Publishing Co, 1970, p 150.

8

Ann Zuzich

8

5. Fletcher J: Situation Ethics. Philadelphia, Westminster Press, 1967, pp 60, 95, 135.
6. Chomsky N: The formal nature of language. *In* Lenneberg EH: Biological Foundations of Language. New York, John Wiley & Sons Inc, 1967, pp 397-442.
7. Engelhardt HT: The roots of science and ethics. The Hastings Center Report 6:36, June 1976.

2

Professional Codes and Personal Values: Some Implications of Incongruence

Mary Reardon Castles, R.N., Ph.D.

Nurses who are involved in activities related to the maintenance of health, the prevention of illness, and the care and cure of persons who become ill, deal daily and at concrete and immediate levels with situations requiring value judgments. How the professional purveyors of health behave is of some consequence to society; students are exposed to information and aided in the development of skills which allow them to make those professional decisions which will be of maximum utility either to their patients, to the community, or to the nursing profession. In the clinical curricula, students are taught to identify assessment parameters and utilize treatment modalities in an explicitly value-free manner; that is, they are taught that their personal feelings and values should not affect their professional behaviors. Assumptions concerning the right of every individual to long life, optimal health, and the best of care in illness underlie the philosophies of schools of nursing. Students are encouraged to believe that they are able and required by professional norms to provide nursing which supports these rights, which is not influenced by personal values, and which is provided equally to all persons.

The myth of value-free professional behavior is pernicious in that it allows personal values to remain hidden and practitioners to remain unaware of the effects of unexamined priorities on care.

Personal values do affect professional behaviors and exert a great, if covert, influence on both patient care and teaching activities. In a profession in which the decisions of practitioners have literally life and death implications for clients, attention to values influencing decisions is demanded. How these values may affect choices among alternative actions in, for instance, situations demanding triage, or situations demanding a selection between societal and individual goods, must be made explicit.

Mary Reardon Castles

Two value systems are considered here: personal values — what one thinks, believes, feels as an individual — and professional values — exemplifying the rhetoric of nursing. Sward[1] suggests that:

> ...a personal code shapes one's basic attitudes and actions, but it is the professional code which is expected to provide direction for professional practice. The professional code presents principles which serve as behavioral norms in the appraisal of conduct and relationships in practice. These principles should...be rationally defensible judgments of how one ought to behave.

A personal code derives from the morality of the society, and dictates the values, priorities, relationships, and behavior of an individual member of the society.

There is in this country a great diversity in religion, education, socioeconomic status, ethnic affiliation, and general cultural norms. Since these differences are well represented in nursing, homogeneity is lacking in just those elements which dictate the formation of personal codes; there is no personal moral consensus shared among nurses, but there is a shared professional code.

A professional code provides public evidence of the values and priorities of a profession. Members are expected to abide by the code, and the profession is expected to take action when they do not. In this way, the code functions as an instrument of accountability to individual clients and to society.

The revised (1976) Code for Nurses[2] makes eleven statements covering several areas of responsibility and obligation including: the obligation to respect human dignity and individuality, to safeguard patients and the public from a variety of threats, to assist in quality assurance activities, to collaborate with other health professionals, to maintain competencies, and to contribute to the professional body of knowledge. Presumably it guides and even dictates decisions relevant to specific practice problems.

In this paper, portions of the first three items of the Code dealing with the provision of services unrestricted by client variables *(item one);* client rights of privacy and confidentiality *(item two);* client safety *(item three);* and the establishment of employment conditions conducive to quality care *(item nine)* are considered.

Decision making is intrinsic to the professional role, and decisions related to professional behavior should be based primarily on the shared professional code, rather than on individual personal values. Since there is diversity in the nursing constituency, deviations from the professional

Professional Codes and Personal Values

code in response to differing personal values would allow nurses' behavior to be unpredictable, and therefore stressful to patients. Indeed, it is difficult to fault the dictates of the Code, which implements an obviously humanistic intent.

The introduction points out that while all situations cannot be anticipated, items are widely applicable and, together with the gloss provided for each item, "provide a framework for the nurse to make ethical decisions and discharge responsibilities to the public, to other members of the health team, and to the profession." The introduction indicates the personal obligation of each nurse to adhere to the Code, and to insure that colleagues also do so. The preamble describes both nurses and clients as individuals and groups "who possess basic rights and responsibilities and whose values and circumstances command respect at all times." The Code is to provide guidance in carrying out nursing responsibilities "consistent with the ethical obligations of the profession and quality in nursing care." It is explicit in demanding that while nurses are carrying out nursing functions, they should be in compliance with its dictates, although respect for the personal values of the practitioner is explicit throughout. Consideration for personal values which may conflict with the professional statement is to be found in the preamble and in the gloss to *item one* which states that although the provision of care is not limited by personal attitudes or beliefs, the nurse can refuse to participate if she is personally opposed to the delivery of care because of the nature of the problem, or the procedure to be carried out. She is, however, held responsible for advance notice of her refusal to deliver care, so that other arrangements for care can be made. In an emergency, or when she is drawn into a situation unknowingly, "the obligation to provide the best possible care is observed." She withdraws only when she is assured care will be provided without her. The professional value takes precedence; the personal value may not be dysfunctional to the quality of nursing care.

It is instructive to examine the guidelines which might be provided by the Code for two common nursing decisions: the decision of what kinds of care shall be given to whom, and in what order (the triage function), and the decision to prescribe or implement placebo therapy.

Item one indicates that the nurse provides services with respect for human dignity, unrestricted by considerations of socioeconomic status, personal attributes, or the nature of the health problem. The interpretative paragraphs accompanying this item *(1.2; 1.3; 1.5)* speak to

Mary Reardon Castles

the principle of non-discriminatory, nonprejudicial care: whoever the individual and whatever his background and circumstances, his nursing care should be determined solely by his human needs, and should not be limited by the setting.

While nurses would agree that care is best determined by human need, the assumption in the statement is that there are adequate resources to provide all of the required services. Such an ideal circumstance would at the least cause comment; it is much more likely that nurses are required to ration inadequate resources in some reasonably equitable manner. Since the requirement of the Code is for care dictated by need, personal values come into play when triage decisions must be made.

An example of the necessity for triage and the variables which may be considered in the unequal allocation of resources is found in the programs developed for patients with end stage renal disease. Under the provisions of *Section 299-1* of *Public Law 92-603,* 90-95% of patients with renal disease who require hemodialysis or transplants are eligible for Medicare, which pays 90% of their costs.[3] Dialysis is, in effect, financially available to everyone, and without treatment patients will die. However, many teams now question whether dialysis should be utilized in all cases. The active collaboration required from dialysis patients in order for treatment to succeed is more likely to be present in people from certain social groups; characteristics likely to be present in middle class, educated persons are important variables in compliance with the rigorous therapeutic requirements, and active, even enthusiastic compliance with the arduous regimen is necessary for successful treatment. In spite of the astronomical sums of money spent on the program, there continue to be more patients than there are available openings. How should selection be made in the face of equal need? Certainly there are medical, social, and psychological variables which can be considered in the allocation equation, but how are they to be weighted? Should an elderly woman with heart disease who has a strong wish to live (a possible indicator of cooperation with the regimen) be denied access to treatment in order that a depressed young man with a family be accommodated? Is value to the community a relevant consideration, and if it is, who defines levels of community value, and what guidelines should be utilized in the definition? Even if institutions refer such questions to ethics committees, personal rather than professional values must be utilized in the decisions.

Conflict in the rights of individuals necessarily leading to triage, which is more clearly and specifically nursing triage responsibility, can be found in the decisions of a night duty charge nurse on a division housing several seriously ill persons. In order to accommodate the victims of a multiple automobile crash in the intensive care unit, several persons are moved from the ICU to her division. What are her options in the face of general need and short staffing, if she wishes to adhere to the mandates of her professional code? Does she mobilize the best resources of the division around the life support needs of one or two severely damaged persons? Does she do the best she can for the many, ignoring the greater needs of one or two? Does she do an excellent best for a reasonable number, shorting the many somewhat, and not providing nearly enough for the sickest persons? Obviously equality of care is not feasible, nor is the determination of care by human needs. Some form of triage is necessary when demand exceeds supply; personal values will play a major and usually unexplored part in the decisions (as, of course, will system constraints, although that is not addressed here).

In addition to the nondiscriminatory mandate of the gloss, the first item *(1.1)* in the code[2] speaks to the self-determination of clients, their involvement in planning their care, their right to be given the information necessary for making informed judgments, and to be told the possible effects of care. Although one paragraph of the interpretation suggests that the nurse must recognize those situations in which individual rights to self-determination in health care may be *temporarily* altered for the common good (emphasis mine), paragraph one certainly appears to rule out the use of placebos, a therapy which is endorsed almost unanimously by clinical prescribers as being in the best interests of patients. In this situation, the Code does *not* mandate what is usual practice, and the conflict lies in the difference between the official expression of a value and practice. The conflict can be further confounded if personal values do not allow that competent adults can be deceived for their own good. Surely it is a deception if the nurse tells the patient his pain will be relieved by the administration of an inert substance rather than the analgesic or narcotic the patient expects. Although the nurse may truly believe the patient will experience relief of pain, and he may do so, the intention is certainly to deceive since deception is the basis of the expected good result.

In a further interpretation of *item one (1.6),* the nurse is directed to protect basic values while working with the client and others to arrive at the best decisions allowed by the circumstances, the client's rights and wishes, and the highest standards of care. This is addressed to the care of

Mary Reardon Castles

the dying person. The language allows a stunning variety of patterns of therapy. One such pattern is exemplified by Dr. Haemmerli's "best decisions."[4] He and his staff work in a hospital in Switzerland; many of the patients are elderly and, as a result of cardiovascular accident, lapse into coma. Cerebral function is irreversibly failed, but the deeper brain structures continue operative, so spontaneous respiration continues. These patients are kept alive by artificial feeding through nasogastric tubes. When there is staff consensus that in a certain patient coma is irreversible, the nutrients may be discontinued and the patient given only a solution of salt and water to prevent dehydration; death usually occurs within a few weeks. It is, in fact, death by starvation. It is (as far as anyone knows) painless to the comotose patient. After the staff members make the collective decision to discontinue nutrition, the doctor talks with the family. However, the decision remains a staff decision. The value expressed here is that therapy which is not likely to succeed is pointless; Haemmerli suggests that prolongation of life possibly should not constitute the overriding purpose of medical practice, although the medical rhetoric generally supports this purpose. Haemmerli was brought to trial, acquitted, and continued to prescribe saline feedings. The Swiss Academy of Medical Sciences has now issued guidelines to doctors regarding the cessation of life-prolonging treatment for dying or comotose patients. The four point directive indicated that "renunciation of treatment or its limitation to alleviate sufferings is medically justified if putting off death would mean for the dying an unreasonable prolongation of suffering and if the basic condition has taken...an irreversible course."*

This physician's personal values now begin to be reflected in his professional code, but there still may be a question for the nurses who feed saline instead of nutrients.[5] What is the obligation of nurses to patients in irreversible coma? Historically, and this is reflected in the ANA Code, nurses are patient advocates, patient protectors. The question is whether the patients are to be protected from those physicians and family members who wish to sustain physiological life in the apparent absence of psychological responses, or whether they are to be protected from those who would allow them or even help them to die. The professional Code is not entirely clear and helpful here, and personal values must dictate decisions.

*London Free Press. *London, Ontario, Canada, 21 April 1977, p 3.*

Professional Codes and Personal Values

The ANA Code directs the nurse to act to safeguard the patient when his care and safety are affected by the incompetent, unethical, or illegal conduct of any person *(item three)*.[2] Does she then interfere when she believes the medical statement to the patient is incomplete, inaccurate, or biased in favor of a radical treatment? The nurse who espouses feminist values may experience some difficulty in a situation in which the surgeon has indicated to the patient that radical mastectomy is the best treatment for breast cancer, in view of some of the simple mastectomy survival statistics currently being reported. By the time the initial actions and follow-up actions described by the Code are taken in such a situation, the operation is over, and if there is to be damage to the patient, it has occurred. In any case, the dilution of the patient's trust in the physician may not be an absolute good. Similar conflicts may also be elicited by the implications of the statement in *item nine* identifying the responsibility of the nurse to "participate in the professions' efforts to establish and maintain conditions of employment conducive to high quality nursing care," particularly for those elder nurses who have been socialized in a tradition of service to the patient and to the doctor, regardless of pay, prestige, or staffing patterns. The whole idea of collective action which might include the necessity for interference in the patient-doctor relationship, or the necessity to walk out on present patients in an effort to improve the care of future patients, threatens ingrained values, the examination of which may be extremely painful.

Difficulties also arise in situations in which the rights of individuals conflict with the rights of society. There is an undoubted professional commitment to keep confidential information obtained during the patient-nurse interaction *(item two);* but if during a home visit to a post-partal patient a transaction involving the exchange of money and marijuana is perceived by the nurse, what is to be kept confidential? Is there a citizen responsibility to report a crime which overrides the nursing responsibility to keep a patient confidence? Is the incident to be considered merely as part of the environmental assessment parameter which will influence the care plan? If the exchange involved hard drugs, does this influence the decision to report? The contributions of the professional code to such decisions is not clear. It does not indicate how to resolve conflict between professional and personal values nor how to resolve conflict over changing values in the profession and in society.

Difficulties arise when components of the professional code exclude personal values, and when practice activities do not reflect the dictates of

Mary Reardon Castles

the code. Analysis of the ethical bases of professional decisions is as important as analysis of the clinical factors, and more difficult to perform. Identification of the conflicts which necessarily arise in a heterogeneous population functioning under a single official code may prevent those conflicts from generating further divisions in nursing.

References

1. Sward KM: The code for nurses: a guide for ethical nursing practice. J NYSNA 4:25-32, 1975.
2. American Nurses' Association: Code For Nurses With Interpretive Statements. Kansas City, Missouri, 1976, pp 1-6, 8, 16.
3. Perkoff G et al: Long term dialysis programs: new selection criteria, new problems. Hastings Center Report 6:8-13, 1976.
4. Culliton BJ: The Haemmerli affair: is passive euthanasia murder? Science 190:1271-1275, 1975.
5. International Council of Nurses Code for Nurses. Geneva, Imprimeries Populaires, 1973.

Bibliography

Bok S: The ethics of giving placebos. Scientific American 231:17-23, 1974.
Epstein LC, Lasagna L: Obtaining informed consent. Arch Intern Med 123:682-688, 1969.
Fletcher J: Indicators of humanhood: a tentative profile of man. Hastings Center Report 2:1-4, 1972.
Illich I: Medical Nemesis. New York, Pantheon Books, 1976.
Mills DH: Whither informed consent. JAMA 229:305-310, 1974.
Rachels J (ed): Moral Problems. New York, Harper and Row Pubs Inc, 1971.

3

Moral Development: Theory and Process

Darimell Waugh, R.N., M.S.N.

"And the moral of the story is..." Does that sound familiar? How many fables or fairy tales have you read that concluded with a moral lesson? If you read fairy tales as a child, you probably learned very little about the specific conditions of your life, but you probably did learn something about the inner problems of man and about solutions to basic human predicaments in any society. Children have always been enchanted by and have found meaning in fairy tales. By implication, they contribute to the moral education of the child by conveying the advantages of moral behavior, not through abstract ethical concepts but through that which seems tangibly right and, therefore, has meaning for him. "And the moral of the story is..." The tales carry moral messages to the child's conscious, preconscious, and unconscious mind on whatever cognitive level these are functioning.*

There is a disinclination, on the part of adults, to let children know that the source of much that goes wrong in today's society is due to man's nature. We want children to believe that men are inherently good. But every child knows that he is not always good and sometimes even when he is, he would prefer not to be. There is good in every bad little boy as there is bad in every good little girl.

Roots of Kohlberg's Theory

My goal is to present Kohlberg's Theory of Moral Development in a framework that will have meaning and applicability to your areas of function. Dr. Lawrence Kohlberg, an eminent Developmental Psychologist, began to elaborate back in 1955 his typological scheme which

*Bettleheim B: Reflections — the uses of enchantment. New Yorker, 8 December 1975, p 50.

describes general structures and forms of moral thought. Kohlberg's theory aims at giving a structure to lean on, a framework on which to build moral judgment. This structure can be helpful in examining the moral decisions other people make which many may find personally questionable. This structure can also give us an idea of our own personal level of maturity. The "vogue" or the "in" thing to do today is to examine one's "roots" — one's ancestry. Therefore, let us examine the roots of Kohlberg's work as well as the roots of philosophical thought on man's morality. Historically, philosophical thought on man's morality dates back to the days of Socrates and Plato. Socrates was a man who devoted himself completely to seeking truth and goodness. He believed that man's nature leads him to act correctly and in agreement with knowledge and that man's evil and wrong actions arise from ignorance and the failure to investigate why people act as they do. Socrates accepted the penalty of death rather than abandon his devotion to truth.

Plato, a disciple of Socrates, provided us with much of the insight into Socrates' life and teachings through his dialogues. Many of Plato's dialogues try to identify the nature or essence of some philosophically important notion by defining it. The central question of Plato's Republic is "What is Justice?" Plato believed that if a man has the knowledge that moral virtue leads to happiness, he naturally acts virtuously. Thus for Plato, the basic problem of ethics is a problem of knowledge. He also argued that the human soul is divided into three parts: (1) the rational part or intellect, (2) the will, and (3) the appetite or desire. In a properly functioning soul, the intellect — the highest part — should control the appetite — the lowest part — with the aid of the will.

Rousseau was one of the formulators of the philosophical doctrine of "innate purity." In this doctrine, great emphasis is placed on the role of higher mental processes in moral development. Society, especially adult society, is held to be a primarily corrupting influence that should be minimized, especially in the child's early years. A present day representative of Rousseau's is Jean Piaget, director of the institute in Geneva that bears Rousseau's name.[1]

Piaget was also inspired by John Dewey. Dewey stated for the first time the cognitive-developmental approach to moral education. Dewey's theoretical approach is called cognitive because it recognizes that moral education, like intellectual education, has its basis in stimulating the active thinking processes of the child. The approach is developmental because it sees the aims of moral education as movement through stages.

Moral Development: Theory and Process

We give credit to Piaget for his pioneering efforts to define stages of moral reasoning in children through actual interviews and through observations of children in games with rules. In synthesizing his studies of cognitive stages, as well as through use of his interview data, Piaget further defined the cognitive-developmental model.[2] His model takes into account the qualitative change in the individual during the development of the cognitive processes as well as the necessity for an adequately stimulating environment. According to Piaget, it is only natural give and take that occurs in social interactions among peers that can provide the impetus to moral maturity, meaning that morality is guided in the main by higher cognitive processes.[1]

Accepting the basic cognitive-developmental approach of Dewey-Piaget, Kohlberg has redefined, validated, and retained the best of the Dewey-Piaget model in developing his six stages of moral development, and fit it into a more refined, comprehensive, and logically consistent framework.[2] For 12 years, he followed the same group of boys following their development at three year intervals from early adolescent through young manhood. In addition, Kohlberg has explored moral development in other cultures — Canada, Britain, Israel, Taiwan, Yucatan, Honduras, and India.[3]

Rationale for Theory

Kohlberg bases his approach largely upon maturity of moral reasoning. Since maturity of moral reasoning is only one factor in moral behavior, Kohlberg states the following rationale for his thinking:[2]

1. Moral judgment, while only one factor in moral behavior, is the single most important or influential factor yet discovered in moral behavior.

2. While other factors influence moral behavior, moral judgment is the only distinctively moral factor in moral behavior. Will becomes an important factor in moral behavior, but is not distinctively moral. Will becomes moral only when informed by mature moral judgment.

3. Moral judgment change is long range or irreversible; a higher stage is never lost. Moral behavior as such is largely situational and reversible or "loseable" in new situations.

Since moral reasoning clearly is reasoning, advanced moral reasoning depends upon advanced logical reasoning. A person's logical stage puts a certain ceiling on the moral stage he can attain. One cannot follow moral

Darimell Waugh

FIGURE 3-1*
Moral Development: Nature and Process

DILEMMA WORKSHEET I

Reaction

Dilemma: Lita and Amy are best friends and senior nursing students at College A. Last quarter, Lita, pressured by many assignments, decided to purchase from a writer's service her term paper required for one of her nursing courses. The paper counted for 60% of the "A" grade Lita received. Amy is aware of Lita's purchase of the paper and can prove it. During one of their clinical experiences, Lita observes Amy drop an infant on the floor. The infant cries but does not appear hurt. Amy decides not to report the incident. She also tells Lita that if she says anything, she will reveal Lita's term paper purchase. What are Lita's options?

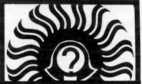

Suggested Resolutions:

_____   _____

_____   _____

_____   _____

_____   _____

_____   _____

_____   _____

_____   _____

_____   _____

_____   _____

_____   _____

*Adapted from "How Moral Am I?" Copyright © 1973 by William H. Sadlier, Inc.

Moral Development: Theory and Process

principles if one does not comprehend moral principles. However, one can reason logically in terms of moral principles and, depending upon the individual's motives and emotions, not live up to these principles. Therefore, mature moral judgment is a necessary but not sufficient condition for mature moral action. Kohlberg's interest as he validated his stages was not in the action alternatives selected by subjects in conflict situations, but in the quality of their judgments as indicated in the reasons given for their choices and their ways of defining the conflict situation.[2]

Before looking specifically at Kohlberg's levels and stages, let us examine a plausible dilemma. After reading Dilemma Worksheet I — Reaction — Lita's Dilemma, suggest one or two possible resolutions to the dilemma in the space provided. (20 minute activity.)

Concept of Stages

To understand moral stages, it is necessary to clarify the concept of stages as used by Piaget and Kohlberg and list how Kohlberg's theory satisfies the characteristics that have been demonstrated for stages. (see page 22.)

Kohlberg's Theory

Kohlberg's theory is divided into three levels of moral thinking. The first level is *preconventional,* the second, *conventional,* and the third, *postconventional.* Within each of these levels, there are two discernible stages.†

Preconventional: At this level, the child is responsive to cultural rules and labels of good and bad, right or wrong, but interprets these labels either in terms of the physical or the hedonistic consequences of action (punishment, reward, exchange of favors) or in terms of the physical power of those who enunciate the rules and labels. This level is usually occupied by children aged four to ten. "Properly behaved children" of this age have the capacity to engage in cruel behavior when there are holes in the power structure. The motive is to avoid external punishment, obtain rewards, have favors returned.

---

†*Excerpted from* Psychology Today Magazine. *Copyright © 1968 Ziff-Davis Publishing Company.*

Darimell Waugh

Concept of Stages	Kohlberg's Stages
1. Stages are "structural wholes" or organized systems of thought. Individuals are *consistent* in level of moral judgement.	1. In validating his stages, Kohlberg found that more than 50% of an individual's thinking is always at one stage with the remainder at the next adjacent stage (which he is leaving or which he is moving into).
2. Stages form an invariant sequence. Under all conditions except extreme trauma, movement is always forward, never backward. Individuals never skip stages: movement is always to the next stage up. The individual proceeds as age and maturational level progress and as the necessary stimulus is provided in the environment.	2. Invariant Sequence — On every retest of subjects, they were found to be at the same stage as three years earlier or had moved up.
3. Stages are hierarchial integrations. Thinking at a higher stage includes or comprehends within it lower stage thinking. There is a tendency to function at or prefer the highest stage available.	3. Kohlberg demonstrated that adolescents exposed to written statements at each of the six stages comprehend or correctly put in their own words all statements at or below their own stage but fail to comprehend any statements more than one stage above their own. Some individuals comprehend the next stage above their own; some do not. Adolescents prefer the highest stage they can comprehend.[2]

Moral Development: Theory and Process

Conventional: At this level, maintaining the expectations of the individual's family, group, or nation is perceived as valuable in its own right, regardless of immediate or obvious consequences. The attitude is not only one of conformity to personal expectations and social order, but of loyalty to it, of actively maintaining, supporting, and justifying the order, and of identifying with the persons or group involved in it. This level can be described as conformist, but perhaps that is too smug a term. The definition of good and bad goes beyond mere obedience to rules and authority. Though control of conduct is external (standards conformed to are rules and expectations held by those who are significant, others by virtue of personal attachment or delegated authority), motivation is largely internal.

Postconventional, Autonomous, or Principled Level: This level is unlike the previous ones in that the possibility of conflict between two socially accepted standards is acknowledged and attempts at rational decision between them are made. Control of conduct is internal in two senses: the standards conformed to have an internal source, and the decision to act is based on an inner process of thought and judgment concerning right and wrong. Moral principles have validity and application apart from authority of the groups or persons who hold them and apart from the individual's identification with those persons or groups.

1. *Preconventional*
   Stage 1: Obedience — Punishment Orientation
   In the first stage the person's behavior is mainly governed by an unquestioning deference to superior power. The Stage-One person does not question this power; his concern is avoiding punishment. The physical effects of an action determine whether it is a good or a bad act regardless of the human meaning or value of these consequences. For instance, a child may not cheat in a game with his big brother because of what his brother may do to him if he is caught. He does not avoid cheating because he values honest behavior. The Stage-One person thinks it is okay to cheat as long as you do not get caught.
   Stage 2: Personal Interest Orientation
   The Stage-Two person is slightly more developed. He considers right action to be anything which satisfies his personal needs, or

sometimes the needs of others. Human relations are viewed in terms like those of marketplace. The Stage-Two person will scratch your back if you'll scratch his, as is standard in business practice. Reciprocity is not a matter of loyalty, gratitude, or justice. Self-satisfaction is parmount, but give and take assumes a role. The Stage-Two person is willing to share equally with another person, but for his own sake. He has begun to develop a sense of fairness, but for practical, pragmatic reasons. He does not grasp yet the universal principle of justice for all men. His concern is still primarily with getting his share.

2. *Conventional*

Stage 3: Good Boy — Nice Girl Orientation

At the conventional level, the Third-Stage person's behavior is oriented toward pleasing others. His concern is finding acceptance. He earns approval by being nice. There is much conformity to stereotypical images of what is majority or "natural behavior." The important rule of behavior for the Third-Stage person is his intention. Even though he may be a bungler, the important thing is that he means well. Behavior is often judged by intention. This becomes important for the first time. In a word, the Stage-Three person is a conformer. This stage prepares the way for a more developed social sense.

Stage 4: Law and Order Orientation

The Stage-Four person's behavior focuses on doing one's duty. The individual is loyal to existing authority. He obeys the laws and promotes keeping the established order. He finds self-respect in fulfilling his obligations. His level of respect for others is based upon their ability to contribute to the established system for its own sake. He may admit that the existing system may have flaws, but only because everyone is not doing his duty.

3. *Postconventional*

Stage 5: Social Contract Orientation

At the postconventional level, we find a more developed moral behavior emerge. The Stage-Five person begins to describe right action in terms of general individual rights and standards which have been critically examined and agreed upon by the whole society. Aside from what is constitutionally and democratically agreed upon,

Moral Development: Theory and Process

the right is a matter of personal values and opinions. The Stage-Five person carries with him some of his Stage-Four sensitivities about one's duty toward the system. But now he works not simply to maintain the status quo; he may work to change the law for the sake of society. Emphasis is upon the "legal point of view" but an orientation to the possibility of changing law in terms of rational considerations of social utility rather than freezing it in terms of Stage Four "law and order." So the Stage-Five person's level of moral thinking is oriented toward majority rule. Outside the legal realm, free agreement and contract is the binding element of obligation.

Stage 6: Conscience Orientation

In the sixth stage of moral development, the person makes decisions of conscience and is guided by self-chosen ethical principles. These principles are abstract; they are not concrete moral rules like the Ten Commandments. He holds these principles even if it means going against the rule of the majority. The Stage-Six person operates according to universal principles of justice — the equality of human rights and respect for the dignity of human beings as individual persons. Consider, for example, the Stage-Six person's explanation of behavior concerning the worth of human life: A person may steal medicine to give it to someone who would die without it. The value of human life is greater than financial gain. The Stage-Six person has become progressively disentangled from property values or social standing. This person shows the greatest capacity for moral behavior.

After hearing about these stages, one cannot help but wonder what stage he is at personally. It should be pointed out that a person who is capable of Stage-Six behavior may not operate at that level in all of his actions. Let us briefly go over the six stages for the sake of clarity:

At Stage-One, avoidance of punishment and deference to power are ends in themselves and form the basis for moral decisions.

At Stage-Two, the necessity to satisfy one's own needs, sometimes the needs of others, forms the basis for moral decisions. He seeks rewards.

At Stage-Three, that which pleases or helps others and is approved by them forms the basis for moral decisions. The Stage-

Darimell Waugh

Three person tries always to be nice.

At Stage-Four, obeying rules and authority, doing one's duty, and maintaining the social order becomes the basis for moral decisions.

At Stage-Five personal values and opinions are regarded as the basis for moral decisions. The Stage-Five person is guided by standards critically examined and agreed to by society.

At Stage-Six, the universal principles of justice, of reciprocity and equality of human rights, and of respect for the dignity of human beings as individuals become the basis for moral decisions.

Each developmental stage is a better cognitive organization than the one before it — one which takes account of everything present in the previous stage, but making new distinctions and organizing them into a more comprehensive or more equilibrated structure. Movement to higher stages of moral development is advantageous not only for the individual but for the society in which he lives. In health care, we often confront moral situations which represent moral dilemmas. Are we preparing ourselves or our students to make the moral choices we are confronted with to the advantage of self, the profession, and the society in which we live?

To conclude, keep in mind that a person operates at a variety of levels. However, fifty percent of most people's thinking will be at a single stage regardless of the moral dilemma involved. A person advances from one stage to another sequentially. The stages represent an invariant sequence. They come one at a time and always in the same order. Children may move through these stages at varying speeds and may be found half in and half out of a particular stage. An individual may stop at any given stage and at any age, but if he continues to move, he must move in accord with these steps.[3]

To complete the activity initiated earlier when you were requested to suggest resolutions to Lita's dilemma, now identify the resolutions you chose in terms of the stages or moral development as defined by Kohlberg.

The second sheet lists various resolution behaviors Lita could have chosen according to each stage of moral maturity.

Moral Development: Theory and Process

FIGURE 3-2**

DILEMMA WORKSHEET II

Analysis

Dilemma: _____

_____

_____

_____

_____

Kohlberg's Stages:

1. Obedience-punishment
   orientation

   Decide so as to avoid
   punishment

2. Personal interest orientation

   Decide so as to satisfy personal
   needs, sometimes needs of
   others

3. Good-boy, good-girl orientation

   Decide so as to please others

4. Authority and social-order-
   maintaining orientation

   Decide so as to maintain
   system

5. Social contract orientation

   Decide so as to further the good
   of the society or
   community

6. Conscience orientation

   Decide so as to sustain personally significant universal
   human principles

Reflections on original resolutions of dilemma (from WORKSHEET 1)
in light of the six stages of moral development:

_____   _____

_____   _____

_____   _____

_____   _____

***Adapted from "How Moral Am I?" Copyright © 1973 by William H.
Sadlier, Inc.*

Darimell Waugh

FIGURE 3-3‡

Lita's Dilemma

Dilemma: Lita and Amy are best friends and senior nursing students at College A. Last quarter, Lita, pressured by many assignments, decided to purchase from a writer's service her term paper required for one of her nursing courses. The term paper counted for 60% of the "A" grade Lita received. Amy is aware of Lita's purchase of the paper and can prove it. During one of their clinical experiences, Lita observes Amy drop an infant on the floor. The infant cries but does not appear hurt. Amy decides not to report the incident. She also tells Lita that if she says anything, she will reveal Lita's term paper purchase. What are Lita's options?

STAGE OF MORAL MATURITY	LITA MIGHT REPORT THE INCIDENT IF SHE FELT	LITA MIGHT NOT REPORT THE INCIDENT IF SHE FELT
I. Obedience-punishment orientation Decide so as to avoid punishment	that the punishment she would receive for purchasing the term paper, should such be revealed, would be less severe than what she could expect from not reporting a patient incident.	a greater fear for the punishment for purchase of the term paper.
II. Personal interest orientation Decide so as to satisfy personal needs, sometimes needs of others.	that she might be able to work out a deal with the faculty concerning her term paper and she would be rewarded (little or no punishment) for "telling the truth."	that her own position would be better served by remaining silent (ie, to trade her silence about Amy's action for silence about her term paper purchase).

III. Good-boy, good-girl orientation Decide so as to please others	that her worth in the eyes of her family, friends, and faculty would be lessened by not reporting the incident.	that avoiding offense to her parents and peers is more important than seeing justice done for the infant.
IV. Authority and social-order-maintaining orientation Decide so as to maintain system	that reporting the incident is the "right" thing to do and that otherwise Amy would "get away" with a violation of rules.	that the informal "code of honor" among fellow students at school would not allow her to inform on Amy and that maintaining the code is more important than seeing justice done.
V. Social contract orientation Decide so as to further the good of the society or community.	that the professional or community's standards of justice and fair play requires that she expose Amy and protect the infant.	if Lita is acting in accord with Stage Five or Six morality, it seems that she would be compelled to tell the truth in order to see society's and/or professional standards upheld and to satisfy her own conscience.
VI. Conscience orientation Decide so as to sustain personally significant universal human principles.	that to protect the individual human rights of the innocent (the infant) would be more important than any personal difficulties she might face, and that her conscience would give her no rest if she allowed the infant's health to be jeopardized.	

Darimell Waugh

References

1. Hoffman M: Moral development. *In* Carmicheal: Manual of Child Psychology, ed 3. New York, John Wiley & Sons Inc, vol 2, pp 261-359.
2. Kohlberg L: The cognitive-developmental approach to moral education. The Humanist 32:12-18, November-December 1972.
3. Kohlberg L: The child as a moral philosopher. Psychol Today 2:28, 1968.

4

Teaching Values: Theory and Process

Dorothy E. Reilly, R.N., Ed.D., F.A.A.N.

RECALLED FOR REVISION
by William C. Miller
Edsel Memorial High School
Anywhere, U.S.A.

Dear Parents of Our Graduates:

As you are aware, one of your offspring was graduated from our high school this June. Since that time it has been brought to our attention that certain insufficiencies are present in our graduates, so we are recalling all students for further education.

We have learned that in the process of the instruction we provided we forgot to install one or more of the following:

at least one salable skill;
a comprehensive and utilitarian set of values;
a readiness for and understanding of the responsibilities of citizenship.

A recent consumer study consisting of follow-up of our graduates has revealed that many of them have been released with defective parts. Racism and materialism are serious flaws and we have discovered they are a part of the makeup of almost all our products. These defects have been determined to be of such magnitude that the model produced in June is considered highly dangerous and should be removed from circulation as a hazard to the nation.

Some of the equipment which was in the past classified as optional has been reclassified as standard and should be a part of every product of our school. Therefore, we plan to equip each graduate with:

a desire to continue to learn;
a dedication to solving problems of local, national, and international concern;
several productive ways to use leisure time;
a commitment to the democratic way of life;
extensive contact with the world outside the school;
experience in making decisions.

In addition, we found we had inadvertently removed from your child his interest, enthusiasm, motivation, trust, and joy. We are sorry to report that these items have

Dorothy Reilly

*been mislaid and have not been turned in at the school Lost and Found Department.
If you will inform us as to the value you place on these qualities, we will reimburse
you promptly by check or cash.*

*As you can see, it is to your interest, and vitally necessary for your safety and the
welfare of all, that graduates be returned so that these errors and oversights can be
corrected. We admit that it would have been more effective and less costly in time
and money to have produced the product correctly in the first place, but we hope
you will forgive our error and continue to respect and support your public schools.*

     Sincerely,

     P. Dantic, Principal*

Should a similar letter be sent to employers of graduates from your
programs? Is there a potential that your students may be hazardous to the
nation? Is a recall in order? These questions are not raised lightly, for they
are intended to make us ponder about what we really have been teaching
our developing practitioners. Principal P. Dantic is stating that the defect
is in the affective domain of learning.

Meaning of Affective Domain in Nursing

What do we mean by the affective domain of learning? Affective
domain is the emotional learning outcome, the feeling tone that is
expressed by such terms as attitudes, beliefs, values, appreciations, or
interests. It is that part of man through which he expresses the self; it is
often the motivation of his behavior. It is an integral part of any decision
that is made. It is a sphere of learning with its own defined limits, yet it is
closely related to and often interfaces with the other two domains of
learning, the *cognitive* and the *psychomotor domains.*

Although man is multidimensional and behaves totally, there has been
continued recognition of the distinction between behaviors of cognition
and emotion. Plato in *The Republic* differentiated three components of
the human soul which were considered to have particular functions in the
life of man: knowing, wanting, willing. Since these components
developed separately, they occurred with different strengths in men:

---

*Miller WC: Recalled for revision. Phi Delta Kappan. *Bloomington, Indiana, Phi Delta Kappa,
December 1971.*

Teaching Values: Theory and Process

some were dominated by intellect, some by passion, and some by power quest. This differentiation in the components of man has received varying interpretation by philosophers and psychologists throughout history, but it was not until Freud and the field theorists such as Lewin demonstrated the significance of emotions on learning behavior that the affective domain became recognized as a legitimate concern in the teaching of the young. Until then, affective learning was primarily relegated to the instinctual field and thought to "just happen" to good people.

I wonder if in too many instances affective learning is still perceived as "just happening." As I think back over my long association with nursing education, I do not have to go very far into the past to see that affective learning was perceived to be "caught" by the student with no suggestion of its being developmental, a quality ascribed to the other domains. The student was expected to evidence all these "fine qualities" of the good nurse, but where they came from was not of primary concern to faculty.

Would we be having this workshop in 1970, just seven years ago? I am not sure. I recall working with various faculty groups on curriculum when any mention for affective learning, especially values, was perceived as imposing one's values on the student. It is interesting that there was never expressed a concern for imposing one's cognition or psychomotor skill on a student. Why was such a danger perceived to be inherent in the teaching of values? Of course, the concept is erroneous for one cannot impose one's own learning on other human beings. Remember how Gibran expressed this concept when asked about teaching:

> ...no man can reveal to you ought, but that which lies half asleep in the dawning of your knowledge.
>
> The teacher who walks in the shadow of the temple among his followers, gives not of his wisdom, but rather of his faith and his lovingness.
>
> If he is indeed wise he does not bid you enter the house of his wisdom, but rather leads you to the threshold of your own mind.[1]

It is not suggested here that nursing educators have not given thought to the affective domain of learning, for indeed many school philosophies and objectives have incorporated the affective component; although in some instances, the component was stated in concomitant objectives rather than outcome objectives of the program. The charge being made here is that affective learning was not treated in the same manner as other learning domains; ie, learning experiences and teaching strategies were not proposed, and protocols for evaluation were not developed.

Dorothy Reilly

Need for Affective Domain

What has happened in the past seven years that brings us together for a workshop as this? Events in our society are now convincing educators that the affective domain of learning is not only a crucial component of any program planning which prepares health care providers but it demands the same pedogogical considerations as the other domains. The affective defects in society and especially in professionals serving society's needs have been evidenced as we have been forced to come to grips with the Vietnam War, Watergate, the human rights movement, consumer demands, the greed contaminating many social programs, the change in the meaning of authority, and the pleas of students that education is more than cognitive skills. The true meaning of the expression, "The person who is the nurse is the critical determinant of the quality of nursing care provided," becomes even more significant.

Schein reminds us that changing social values have created new client systems and are calling upon practitioners to rethink professional roles. He states, "The new values call for the professional to be an advocate, to set about to improve society, not merely to service it, to become more socially conscious, to be more an initiator than a responder."[2] Illich states that medical and health care in Western society is counterproductive as "so called health professionals destroy the potential of people to deal with their human weakness, vulnerability and uniqueness in a personal and autonomous way."[3] C. P. Snow sees many living in Western world today without hope, extremely uneasy about the society in which they live. He identifies the pluralistic nature of Western society as a major source of the difficulty, for there exists no code of common assumptions upon which to build a society by generating a common purpose and a compatible form of action. Accepting the premise that we may indeed need to live with moral discontent, he cautions against false hope and challenges us to stop our flight from reason and to use our science, art, and investigative writing to seek an understanding of our human state. He says, "When we have made that start, we may hope to understand a little more about responsibility and what degrees of freedom we really possess and how our natures are built and what we can do with them."[4]

Schein, Illich, and Snow are speaking to nursing educators. They are asking us to use our unique contact with our fellow man to contribute to the development of new knowledge essential for understanding the human state. They are also asking us to prepare our new practitioners with the competencies essential both to serving the human state in a supportive and humane manner and to contributing to the understanding of the nature of that state.

Concept of Learning as Related to Affective Domain

The first consideration in approaching the teaching of the affective domain of learning is to clarify the meaning of the term, *learning*. Learning is generally accepted as a change in behavior resulting from experience. The experience dimension is critical as it differentiates learning behavior change from behavior changes resulting from other phenomena such as maturation, disease, or alterations in body structure. Thus the provision for learning experiences is essential to the attainment of behavioral change resulting from learning. Krathwohl and his colleagues state that as a result of analyses of research of Tyler, Furst, Dressel, and Jacobs, "The evidence suggests that affective behaviors develop when appropriate learning experiences are provided for students much the same as cognitive behaviors develop from appropriate learning experiences."[5]

The primary goal of this educational endeavor is in assisting the learners in the development of values that support a self-identity that is compatible with the responsibilities inherent in the role of a health care provider in a complex ever-changing pluralistic society. Although this statement emphasizes the process of value development, it also infers that there are certain values that are legitimately taught within a nursing curriculum. Since nursing is a helping profession which provides services to people, practitioners must develop values commensurate with man's worth, his rights as defined by natural law and government documents such as the Bill of Rights in the United States Constitution, and the goal of self-fulfillment within the context of society. Care must be exercised to assure that self-fulfillment is not interpreted as "doing my thing" without any societal responsibility. This interpretation leads to hedonistic behavior.

Once the premise is accepted that value development is a legitimate concern of an educational program for nurse practitioners, where do we go for our theory base to guide our teaching? At this time, our knowledge of value development is on uncertain ground. A theory of values must not

Dorothy Reilly

only account for the existence and operation of human values, but must also be predictive of normative standards of morality by making explicit the principles by which actions are considered to be morally justified. Theories are proposed and efforts to validate them are under way, but the science base is not yet determined. As we move into the realm of values, we are concerning ourselves with the super ego which has not been subject to the scientific inquiry that the other two components of man have been, the *id* and the *ego*.

I rely on two authorities for my framework within which to teach values. One is the theory developed by Louis Raths and his colleagues which emphasizes the process of *value development*. The other is the theoretical concepts underlying the work of Krathwohl and his colleagues in developing the taxonomy of *affective learning*. There is much that is similar in the approach proposed by both of these groups. Rath's theory is a teaching theory which helps us look at the process of developing values, while Krathwohl assists us in teaching the process of the internalization of values.

Although the term, values, is defined in numerous ways, in general a value is accepted as something important in life. Raths et al define values as "those elements that show how a person has decided to use his life." The assumption in this value theory and the proposed teaching strategies is that the "Human can arrive at values by an intelligent process of choosing, prizing, and behaving."[6] Since values are derived from an individual's experience and are learned, the essence of the theory is the teaching of values through the skill of critical thinking.

This theory defines values in terms of three processes: *choosing, prizing, acting.*

Choosing	1. Freely
	2. From alternatives
	3. After thoughtful consideration of the consequences of each alternative
Prizing	4. Cherishing, being happy with choice
	5. Willing to affirm the choice publicly
Acting	6. Doing something with the choice
	7. Repeatedly, in some pattern of life

Since this theory stresses *choosing* as the critical process, it accepts the idea that there are valueless individuals, those who have never made a

Teaching Values: Theory and Process

choice for values. The behavior characteristic of value defects support this concept and include:

1. Apathy — no strong values pulling toward actions.

2. Flighty — search for meaning values.

3. Inconsistent — chooses values expressed by latest groups/individuals with whom he was associated.

4. Hesitant — no value base for declaring a position on an issue.

5. Overconforming — lives in and acts according to values of others, especially one in authority.

6. Overdissenting — nagging, trying to find values.

7. Role playing — trying out various values.

Some behaviors or verbal expressions of individuals have suggested, and indeed have been interpreted as, reflecting values. This theory states that there are value indicators with a potential for becoming values, but until all seven criteria are met, a value is not present. These value indicators are identified as (1) goals, purposes; (2) aspirations; (3) attitudes; (4) interests; (5) feelings; and, (6) beliefs. The teacher's responsibility is to recognize these indicators and assist the learner to move them into values when appropriate.

On the basis of this theory, a value may be defined as an operational belief which an individual accepts as his own and serves as a determinant of his behavior.

A word of caution is needed here about the relationship of value and behavior. Not all behavior is value motivated. At a values classification session, I heard the leader state quite enthusiastically, "Every time you act your values are showing." I challenge this declaration and question where needs behavior fits into this concept.

Needs and values are indeed different and so is the deficiency behavior evidenced by each (Fig. 4-2, Deficiency Behaviors). Raths has identified differentiating characteristics for each (Fig. 4-1, Characteristics of Needs and Values).[6]

Needs, too, are strong determinants of behavior and needs must be met before values can be developed. Love as a value cannot be realized as long as the need for love is predominant. You will also note that needs behavior is the type that we generally dislike and makes us most uncomfortable. We refer to it as "acting out" behavior.

Since critical thinking is the major approach to value development in

Dorothy Reilly

FIGURE 4-1†

Characteristics of Needs and Values

NEEDS	VALUES
1. Start with life	1. Start when child becomes conscious that he is different from what he was
2. Push one into action	2. Pull one toward action
3. Ashamed of	3. Cherish
4. Pervasive	4. Selective
5. Strong visceral component	5. Strong intellectual component
6. Met by others	6. Met by self
7. Deficiency behaviors (Fig. 4-2)	7. Deficiency behaviors (Fig. 4-2)

†Developed from Raths LE, Harmin M, Simon SB: Values and Teaching. Columbus, Ohio, Charles E Merrill Co, 1966.

---

this theory, Raths provides us with a third set of characteristic behaviors with which we must work. These behaviors, unrelated to needs or value motivation, are significant of deficiencies in the thinking process itself. The concept of choosing implies that the student will develop skill in divergent thinking, the determination of alternatives, examination of the consequences of each, and the selection of the best. This thinking contrasts with convergent thinking which requires identification of one possible solution to a problem. The key question, "What else is possible?," is seldom raised by the teacher in working with the student's experience in problem solving. (Maybe we are often relieved that the student arrived at an answer. Maybe we are convergent thinkers.)

Value development, however, must incorporate the element of choice in the thinking process and, therefore, divergent thinking is essential. The behavior characteristics of critical thinking deficiency have been identified (Fig. 4-2).

This approach then provides the teacher with three sets of behaviors

FIGURE 4-2**

Deficiency Behaviors

VALUE	NEED	THINKING
1. Apathy	1. Aggression — inappropriate to solution	1. Impulsiveness in action
2. Flighty	2. Withdrawal	2. Being stuck
3. Inconsistency	3. Submission	3. Missing the meaning
4. Hesitancy	4. Psychosomatic illness symptoms	4. Inflexibility of thought
5. Overconforming		5. Making dogmatic statements
6. Overdissenting		6. Fearfulness about thinking
7. Role-playing		7. Wishful thinking

**Developed from Raths LE, Harmin M, Simon SB: Values and Teaching. Columbus, Ohio, Charles E Merrill Co, 1966.*

with which to diagnose the learner's difficulties. It prevents the teacher from the tendency to make inferences about an individual's values from all behavior which is demonstrated. With proper diagnosis, the teacher can then select appropriate strategies to assist the learner as he proceeds with his value development.

The teaching of values, as has become obvious so far, involves not just the affective domain, but also the cognitive domain. Indeed, in some instances value development teaching may also be concerned with the psychomotor domain. This point can well be illustrated with the competency of the psychomotor skill of touch. Think how much expertise in this skill influences the nurses ability to give evidence of a respect for the value of man's dignity and worth.

The value development theory of Raths and his colleagues, however, does not totally satisfy me as a teacher of nursing, for it emphasizes the process of value development irrespective of the values selected by the student. It says, in essence, that the concern is not what value, but rather how the student arrived at the particular value. In nursing the value as it relates to the professional role is important to us.

The concepts underlying the taxonomy of the affective domain developed by Krathwohl and his colleagues help us as teachers to identify the appropriate values and state them as behaviors according to a sequencing which leads to internalization. The plan of the taxonomy is compatible with the value development process theory of Raths and his colleagues. The first two levels relate to value indicators. It is at the third level where choosing occurs and internalization begins. The levels in the taxonomy are:

1. Receiving — an awareness.
2. Responding — reaction to a situation with some satisfaction.
3. Valuing — the stage of choosing and expressing a commitment to act.
4. Organization — the stage of establishing the internalized value into a system evidencing priorities.
5. Characterization by a value or value complex — the degree of internalization wherein the individual is consistent in behavior, formulated his philosophy of life through integration of all affective components.[5]

The value development process as described by Raths et al, and the taxonomy developed by Krathwohl and colleagues, provide a framework for nursing educators to teach the affective component of nursing. The

Teaching Values: Theory and Process

theories and concepts proposed by these two groups are congruent with Kohlberg's Theory of Moral Development which was presented earlier.

How do we use these theories in developing teaching strategies that will help us reach our goal of affective learning? Two elements are present: (1) experience, (2) critical thinking. It is obvious, I am sure, that teaching values by fiat, precept, threat, or promise of external reward is not a part of these theorists' approach.

Teaching by model has been stressed by many educators. In the September 21, 1976, issue of the *New York Times Magazine,* Amitai Etzioni addresses this issue in an article, "Do As I Say, Not As I Do." He expresses concern with the emphasis on various teaching strategies for teaching values when the learner is exposed constantly in the school environment to practices and behaviors which mitigate against the very values being developed in the classroom setting.

There is no doubt that model teaching is a significant method and we learn much through this approach. However, Adelson warns us of the danger of this type of teaching when he differentiates between the teacher's style and the teacher's skill. Too often it is the style that is imitated rather than the skill serving as a model outcome.[7] The same danger may occur in value teaching. The student may emulate the value behavior of the teacher without ever examining the behavior in relation to its rationale and appropriateness for the student himself.

As educators, we too are being required to assess our own value system to determine consistency between action and espousal. I wonder how far along in the affective domain taxonomy each of us is at this point in our lives. Recognizing that our values must be continuously under scrutiny and are not set in cement once the criteria are met, how ready are we to handle inconsistency in our behavior when it occurs relative to those values we profess?

Teaching-Learning Climate

One of the crucial aspects of teaching values is the climate in which the teaching and learning occur. Value development calls for honest searching. It means risk taking — making oneself vulnerable to judgmental perceptions of others — and often "acting out" as the search for the best of fit occurs. These explorations can occur within a climate of authenticity, trust, support, and freedom from unwarranted sanctions.

Dorothy Reilly

These characteristics do not describe a laissez faire setting. Indeed, limits should be defined and areas of accountability identified, for freedom to learn does not suggest a lack of structure. Certainly the clinical practice setting provides our students with an exceptionally fine environment for value development, but it has inherent within its nature a structure within which the student must function. It is not meant here that all the structural limitations are rational, but it is the responsibility of the faculty member to identify the true boundaries and differentiate them from these limits which a professional may transcend with intelligent risk-taking activities.

The teacher and student must be comfortable in the learning environment for value development. They must respect each other; trust each other. They must share a degree of openness that enables growth to occur, for growth is destined for both the teacher and the learner. A teacher must feel comfortable in sharing feelings about own values and supporting a rationale for the choice made. However, it is essential that the faculty encourage the student to pursue own value choices. Assistance from the teacher may be provided by selecting learning experiences which will enable the student to examine the value he is seeking to develop. Some of these experiences may mean confrontation, for the true test often occurs at the time of hard choices between stands on issues that are meaningful to the individual. The search for values is often not an easy process, especially as one reaches the stage where internalization occurs and a commitment is required. The teacher's recognition of the nature of this process and the support necessary as the student is guided through the critical thinking activities enables the learner to reach his goal with a recognition of accomplishment in determining the value as his own.

In preparation for the discussion on specific teaching strategies, it is important to pause a moment to examine the ultimate purpose of our programs. All of us are committed to preparing nursing practitioners who are accountable for providing quality care and who can participate with others at various levels in assuring quality of health care to our citizenry. Maria Phaneuf, in the new edition of her book, *The Nursing Audit: Self-Regulation in Nursing Practice,* challenges us as professionals when she states, "Self-regulation of nursing practice is a manifestation of professional accountability."[8] She reminds us that this self-regulation entails ethical and moral obligations. Are we preparing practitioners with the ethical and moral framework for self-regulating not only their

Teaching Values: Theory and Process

own practice, but the practice of nursing by all members of the profession? It is the teaching of this framework that is our responsibility to our students, agencies, and society. If we do not, then a recall of our graduates will be in order in the not too distant future.

Criteria for Selecting Teaching Strategies

Many of the strategies discussed here are already being used in most nursing programs. Suggestions will be made to extend the parameters of the methods so that the affective focus can be broadened. Remember that there is a close relationship among all domains and that there is an affective counterpart to all cognitive behavior and, certainly in nursing, for all psychomotor behaviors. Thus, the teaching of the affective domain does not occur in isolation and does not call for a whole new course or unit in a nursing program. Much of value teaching will occur concurrently with other teaching, but there may be times when a particular emphasis in the affective component may be indicated.

Two criteria are essential in selecting and using methods for teaching values. They are: (1) *experience* and (2) *critical thinking* Experiences may involve only the student or they may involve the student in interaction with various individuals and groups. Individual experiences may involve such activities as reading, listening to music, visiting art museums and exhibits, painting, writing, exploring various neighborhoods in a community, or using periods of time for reflection or contemplation. How often do we encourage students to examine the literature in an effort to understand more about the nature of man? One student in a course I taught demonstrated through such readings as Lord Jim, Shakespeare's sonnets, and others, how nursing students could learn much about human behavior. Might we not suggest the student examine the arts to see the message of man expressed through these media? What does a ballet or a piece of music tell us? I attended a very exciting session where students played recordings of popular hit tunes for teenagers that vividly portrayed the alienation that many young people were experiencing. A student in graduate school danced her doctoral thesis as she demonstrated the meaning of dance in an African tribe to depict the values of that culture. We could cite many examples, but the medium is the message; so let us use it more.

Group experiences are numerous and provide excellent opportunity for students to explore values. Interactions may be with colleagues in social and professional settings, with faculty, family, clients, community groups, and even with strangers. What values are evident in these groups? What similarities? What differences?

As the teacher has the opportunity to guide the student's group activity and associations, it is important to recognize that value development does not proceed if the student's other person contacts are solely with people whose values and life styles are like his own. The challenge to choose comes when differences are encountered and the student is called upon to take a stand or declare a position. A student whose clinical practice is primarily with clients who share a similar value system, or non-value system, has no opportunity to test his beliefs, values, and attitudes to determine what values he really has chosen for himself.

The second process, critical thinking, must occur regardless of the nature of the experience. A recounting of the experience is not sufficient. An intellectualizing approach is not sufficient. To use the experience for value development, the student must become involved in the experience and not assume the posture of an outsider. Affective behavior is "being." The faculty must be alerted to the student who is an intellectualizer about a value but has not carried the critical thinking process to the point of making a choice. It is in the use of the critical thinking approach that many teaching strategies currently in use can be expanded to incorporate more depth in the teaching of the affective domain.

The critical thinking competency is acquired under the guidance of a skillful teacher. As a diagnostician, the teacher identifies behaviors signifying deficiencies in values, needs, or in the process of critical thinking itself. Appropriate interventions are implemented. The teacher must be particularly alert to behaviors indicating critical thinking difficulties, for skill in this process is essential to value development.

Since critical thinking demands interaction between the principles involved, the teacher must be alert to own behavior. On issues which the teacher tends to value deeply, there may be a tendency to moralize. This approach may not only "turn off" the student, but it also violates the learner's right to explore his own ideas and feelings so that he can arrive at a choice which is his own. Raths warns us, "We must learn that we cannot foster the ability to think critically in value related issues at the same time that we demand, even subtly, that the outcome of that thinking must conform to what we believe."[6]

Since some of us might have difficulty in following this order not to moralize, I will offer you the six suggestions Raths offers to help us:

Teaching Values: Theory and Process

1. With value issues, avoid questions to which you already have an answer in mind.

2. Avoid "why" questions, "yes-no" questions, "either-or" questions, or questions that tend to make a student defensive, ready to rationalize his position, or that limit his choices.

3. Begin with written value lessons so you can reread your responses before students see them.

4. Ask a colleague to listen to your classroom responses or to read your written comments on value issues and to note moralizing tendencies.

5. Ask students if they feel you are loading the dice about issues that you feel are not loaded.

6. In early stages of value teaching strategies, start with topics in which you have no strong feelings. This is particularly important until students feel comfortable in challenging or differing with your perspective.

Teaching Strategies

What teaching strategies are available that provide for both experiencing and critical thinking? Simon and other colleagues of Raths have proposed numerous values clarification strategies that are directed toward helping the learner see what values he has and how he arrived at them. The strategies are designed to assist the students to build the seven valuing processes into their lives. The method relies on critical thinking process. Since there is a source book out on various strategies, they will not be discussed here, but I recommend that you explore these strategies and select ones that would be of interest to you in relation to the behavioral objectives developed for your program or course. However, a word of caution is needed in using these strategies. Their use for conscience-raising is not enough. The goal in any strategy must be the facilitation of the internalization of values compatible with quality of life.

What mechanisms already exist? Group conferences or discussions are excellent means for the sharing of ideas and beliefs as well as providing for vicarious experiencing. Not all group discussions are conducive to value development process. Nouwen sees group discussions as often violent methods of teaching. He perceives that often a discussion is an intellectual battle from which people tend to return more close-minded than when they entered it. His description of the dynamics is as follows:

Dorothy Reilly

...as soon as someone states an opinion, the most common reaction is not the
internal question: "How can I understand his opinion better?" but "What is my
opinion?" So too, does silence often mean more an occasion to prepare an answer
than to enter the train of thought of the other and once two or three or more
opinions are stated, the primary concern becomes defense of the chosen position
even when it is hardly worth defending.[9]

The dynamics of the process as described by Nouwen are not
productive to a critical thinking process. When the group process strategy
is used, the teacher must monitor the process to be sure that the thinking
follows in the appropriate disciplined manner and the alternatives are
evident for all to examine.

The subject matter of these deliberations may be generated from any
experience the student is having within the framework of the program.
Topics may be developed also from experiences occurring outside the
defined program that have a bearing on the professional behavior of
students. The nature of nursing practice lends itself to a dialogue
approach because of its moral and ethical base. The stated objectives help
to focus the content matter, but since every nursing action involves the
affective domain, the opportunities for value teaching through group
methods are endless.

Nursing practice entails enumerable decision making activities, all of
which have both an affective and a cognitive component. Decision
making process by definition entails a divergent thinking whereby one
must choose from alternatives proposed as solutions to the problem.
Faculty who recognize both domains of learning occurring in this
experience will focus questioning and the explanation of the decision
from the value implications as well as the cognitive ones. It is the latter
that receives most attention presently, but the situation is present to
place the same nursing action under the scrutiny of the valuing process.

Role playing has been used quite frequently for the affective domain of
learning. It is a more appropriate method for this learning than for
cognitive learning. However, I am not certain that the critical thinking
process always receives as much emphasis as does the experiencing
dimension. Role playing is an effective strategy for trying out various
value directed approaches to nursing situations provided the critical
thinking process is followed rigorously.

Multimedia offer a vast array of behavior actions which can be explored
for the value connotations. Episodes depicting interactions of nurses with
others, a family or group interactions, and societal events provide for
vicarious experiencing and lend themselves for critical analyses from a

cognitive and an affective perspective. Situations depicted may be interventions, diagnosing process, decision making and communication, or self-explorations of phenomena.

Field trips to environments different from the ones with which the students are accustomed can help the student broaden the base of knowledge necessary for choosing values. Experiences with various cultural foods, lifestyles, recreation, and family relationships are most critical, especially as they relate to the clients with whom the learners are involved.

Exposure to varied value related patterns of behavior and lifestyles within various socioeconomic groups is essential if the student is to choose own values. Again, these experiences must go beyond the experiencing and the report of observations. The student's own involvement must be explored and the value judgments made need to be examined critically. Judgments may reflect stereotypic value assessment of behavior. The learner will need to differentiate behavior that is situational coping with the immediate realities, from cultural behavior that is reflecting values transmitted through the group throughout several generations. If the student is to be helped in developing the necessary data base, then these experiences must be selected on the basis of learning need. Faculty generally feel that the middle- and upper-class students need experience with clients in an inner city or rural depressed area, but is the reverse not also true? Would not students from the inner city or rural area need experience with clients from the middle- and upper-socioeconomic strata of our society?

Clinical practice itself has a boundless wealth of material for the value development process. All activities and interactions have an affective dimension for learning. Selection of learning experiences may be as appropriately made for affective learning needs as for cognitive or psychomotor needs.

I am sure we could think of many more strategies for teaching the affective domain. It is evident from the above discussion that we do not need to develop whole new curriculums and teaching strategies. We need to expand those methods we are currently using to encompass a more concentrated effort to help the student with the value development process. The content has always been there; the experiences have always been available; it is just that we have not taken advantage of the opportunities to teach for affective learning. Perhaps now that the approach has been brought to a state of awareness, we can move forward with this goal.

I refer you to the essay of Marie Czmowski published in *Nursing Forum* called "Value Teaching in Nursing."[10] In this essay, Marie demonstrates the teaching of the value of privacy within a nursing program using many of the teaching strategies with which you are familiar.

References

1. Gibran K: The Prophet. New York, Alfred A. Knopf Inc, 1968, p 56.
2. Schein EH: Professional education: some new directions. Carnegie Commission on Higher Education. New York, McGraw-Hill Book Co, 1972, p 3.
3. Illich I: Medical Nemesis. New York, Pantheon Books, 1976, p 33.
4. Snow CP: Grounds for hope? N Y Univ Quart 7:27, Summer 1976.
5. Krathwohl D, Bloom BS, Masia BB: Taxonomy of Educational Objectives, Handbook II, Affective Domain. New York, David McKay Co Inc, pp 20, 176-185.
6. Raths LE, Harmen M, Simon SB: Values and Teaching. Columbus, Ohio, Charles E Merrill Pub Co, 1966, pp 6, 170-171, 197-200.
7. Adelson J: The teacher as a model. American College. New York, John Wiley & Sons Inc, 1962, p 404.
8. Phaneuf MC: Nursing Audit: Self-Regulation in Nursing Practice, ed 2. New York, Appleton-Century-Crofts, 1976, p 9.
9. Nouwen H: Creative Ministry. New York, Doubleday & Co Inc, 1971, p 7.
10. Czmowski M: Value teaching in nursing. Nurs Forum, vol. 12, no. 2, 1974.

5

Evaluation: Theory and Strategies

Dorothy E. Reilly, R.N., Ed.D., F.A.A.N.

if
you believe in me
then maybe
i can do something worthwhile.....
  maybe i am worthwhile.....
maybe i can do something with my life

thus
the light of hope begins to burn
 your constant trust in me
   communicates warm sensations of confidence
    and faith
that look in your eyes
 the touch of your hands
  brings me some marvellous message of hope

Jean Vanier[1]

How would you evaluate this expression of Jean Vanier? How are you going to quantify the results of your evaluation data? Suppose that a student wrote this in response to an experience with a patient who found the student a source of hope. What would you do with it? How would it fit with other evaluation data you might gather about that particular student?

As I read this particular page in Jean Vanier's book *Tears of Silence,* something happened to me. I felt! This feeling experience was different from my other reading activities. I pondered how, as a teacher, I would respond to a student paper that made me feel rather than primarily stimulate my intellectual processes. How would I evaluate such a paper if it did not fit my correcting code? And heavens, what would I ever do about grading?

The quotation of Jean Vanier cannot be quantified for it is too close to

Dorothy Reilly

human experience. The security of quantifiable data is not readily found in evaluating affective learning. It does not readily lend itself to the American emphasis on objective data, measurability, and quantification.

Affective learning can be evaluated. True, appraisal strategies at this point are crude in contrast to those available for cognitive learning. William James, the noted empiricist psychologist, addressed the issue of the relationship between psychology and teaching in his *Talks to Teachers*.

> I say moreover that you make a great, a very great mistake, if you think that psychology, being the science of the mind's laws, is something from which you can deduce definite programmes and schemes and methods of instruction for immediate schoolroom use. Psychology is a science and teaching is an art, and sciences never generated arts directly out of themselves. An intermediary inventive mind must make the application by using its originality.[2]

Since evaluation is an integral part of teaching, we must heed James' admonition and not rely solely on psychology to provide us with the evaluation protocols. Your inventive mind is being summoned.

Barriers to Evaluating Affective Domain

In preparation for the discussion of the evaluation process as it relates to affective learning, it is important to examine the barriers that have interfered with our development of a systematic approach to evaluation in this domain of learning. To some extent affective learning has been evaluated, for faculty are often aware of students' interests, attitudes, and stated beliefs. Unfortunately, the data base represents the unusual behavior or the most overt behavior which can be readily categorized as good or bad according to the faculty member's perception. Responses to these behaviors tend to be in the realm of reward or punishment and the behaviors are seen as ends in themselves, unrelated to the totality of the learner. A systematic evaluation protocol is needed in affective learning which recognizes its developmental nature and its outcome.

Cognitive learning has received the major emphasis in evaluation because it lends itself most readily to available appraisal techniques. More will be said later about the level of cognitive behavior that is primarily evaluated, however.

Affective learning at one point in time did receive considerable

Evaluation: Theory and Strategies

emphasis under the rubric of character building. The demands of a technological society with its emphasis on facts resulted in much evaluation data being obtained about the student's mastery of facts. Affective learning became de-emphasized. The additional requirement that all evaluative data be collapsed into a single symbol, the grade, precipitated the movement toward data on cognitive learning as the most important measurement of learning because of its easy convertibility to a grade.

Another barrier has been our tendency to dichotomize the nature of man. We perceive his cognitive behavior as a public matter subject to scrutiny, but his affective behavior is perceived to be in the private realm, therefore unavailable for examination by others. Our American emphasis on privacy has denied us the opportunity to examine the process of teaching the affective domain. An effort to teach in this realm is perceived as indoctrination, a process that by its nature denies the element of choice. However, if education is accepted as a process by which free choices are available and then examined in terms of their consequences so that appropriate choices are made, education is not indoctrination.

James describes choices appropriate to the educational experience. "Human freedom does not mean any choices that tempts us, but choices that lead to the maturation of our human capacities."[3]

The development of such choices involves the affective component of man in concert with his cognitive skills. The notion that as educators we can assist learners in making mature choices by evaluation of only one component, the cognitive, is spurious. Every cognitive action has an affective dimension, and every affective response has a cognitive dimension.

Another barrier relates to the perception of time necessary to develop affective learning. Cognitive learning is discerned to be acquired in a relatively short span of time whereas affective learning is deemed to be a long time process. Both types of learning are taxonomized from simple to complex behavior. My observation suggests that in many courses, cognition evaluation is directed primarily to the lower level skills of information recall, comprehension, and application. Since the complex skills of analysis, synthesis, and evaluation are considered to require an extended period of time to develop and are difficult to appraise, they are less likely to appear within the framework of a course.

Evaluation of affective learning within a course is assumed to be

Dorothy Reilly

directed primarily at the complex level, and since that learning level, like the high level of cognition, requires time to develop and requires more sophisticated evaluation strategies, it is deemed impossible to evaluate. If affective learning behaviors were identified at the lower levels of the taxonomy, they too could be more easily appraised.

In essence, for both domains the lower levels of learning behaviors can be evidenced within a reasonable space of time and can be evaluated with rather easily developed appraisal strategies. In both domains, the complex learning behaviors require an extended period for development and require sophisticated appraisal techniques. The level of development to be achieved within any course or program represents professional judgments of the faculty. In general, upper division and graduate nursing courses ought to be concerned with evaluating the complex behavior of both domains.

Concept of Evaluation

Clarification of the concept of evaluation is essential before we discuss various approaches to the evaluation of affective learning, for I feel that each of us here has a private image of the process and there may well be discrepancies in the perceptions of the process.

The sources of this image are as varied as the types of images represented in this room. For some, the image is derived from concepts or theories found in the literature; for others, the image reflects the process as we saw it in operation when we were students; while for others, the image may be more a "gut reaction" representing our needs, values, or expectations. Indeed, with some of us the manner in which we carry out the process reflects a mixture of all three sources. One might ask, "Is there such a thing as a clearly defined process called evaluation of learning?"

Before proceeding to the identification of a concept of the evaluation process, it is important to deal with one matter which often interferes with our ability to explore the dynamics of evaluation. This matter relates to the frequency with which the terms, *evaluation* and *grading,* are used synonymously. Are evaluation and grading the same? There are two aspects of similarity in these two terms; namely, they are both processes and both have something to say about the performance of an individual. However, they are not the same processes. Evaluation is a judgmental process. Teachers make judgments about the quality of the learner's

Evaluation: Theory and Strategies

attainment of designated behavioral objectives. Grading is a quantitative process by which teachers quantify evaluative data and assign symbols that represent the student's level of academic achievement. Evaluation precedes grading. Grading, the quantitative process, depends upon the data supplied by the qualitative process, evaluation. Evaluation may exist as an independent phenomenon while grading must always depend upon evaluation.

Although, as presented here, evaluation and grading are two distinct processes which are sequential, in reality we know that this distinction is not practiced. Grading and evaluation are often treated as synonymous terms. Formal grades have become the most conspicuous means of assessing student performance in spite of the fact that the fidelity with which they translate the evaluation of learner performance is open to question.

Two dichotomous interpretations of the term evaluation are that (1) it is a process for growth or (2) it is a process for control. The implications of these two quite different interpretations cannot be ignored. If we accept the concept of evaluation as a process or a series of processes by which *value judgments* are made about someone's performance, we can see that evaluation indeed may be used according to the desire of the evaluator.

Let us look at the word, evaluation. I previously used the expression, value judgment. The term value is an integral part of the word, e-*value*-ation. Since values are operational beliefs which one accepts as his own and uses as a determinant of his behavior, we can immediately see that there is no such process as objective evaluation, especially for clinical practice; that quest is in vain, for no such phenomenon exists. However, even though evaluation cannot be objective, evaluation can be fair. It is this quality of fairness that must be our goal.

The evaluator's attitude toward evaluation is one of the critical determinants in relation to the use for which this process is directed. Our attitude determines whether we will ask the right questions and will see the right behavior. This matter of attitude is of particular significance in affective learning, for the concern here is the learner's self-development, the internalization of values that are compatible with a professional role and a self-fulfilling life. The feeling component to affective learning makes it particularly vulnerable to attitudes of evaluators. Do our approaches to the process really support the learner's pursuit of self-knowledge?

Dorothy Reilly

My experiences as an educator suggest that in too many instances, the student's pursuit for self-knowledge is deterred by the messages he receives from his evaluators. Evaluation is not viewed as a facilitating process for self-development, but rather as a "checking process" by which the learner may be stamped with some label for life. The learner's approach to evaluation is self-preservation rather than self-actualization.

Indeed, the interpretation of the meaning of the term evaluation that you as an evaluator use will determine the approach you use and the climate you engender. All helping professions attract certain individuals with a need to control other human beings. These "controllers of men" find the service fields a particularly fertile area, for the clients are often individuals or groups in a dependent state. The controllers rely on rules, regulations, and procedures for evaluative judgments and seek to manipulate the learner into the accepted mode of behavior. Learners then direct their energies toward survival in the system rather than toward experiences which contribute to growth and development.

Evaluation often reflects the student's skill in gamesmanship, rather than his ability to meet the expressed objectives of the learning experience. Professional education, which includes a practice component, is particularly vulnerable to this gamesmanship and is fostered by the evaluator who is controller. The very nature of the supervisory process generates many anxieties which differentiate evaluation of clinical practice from the usual academic situation. Competency in clinical practice relates to all domains of learning: cognitive, affective, and psychomotor. Changes in behavior in all these domains occur within the confines of a close relationship with the teacher and often in full view of peers, patients, and other professionals or practitioners. Feelings of inadequacy subject the learner to fears of criticism, shame, and rejection. If the teacher in the clinical setting places value primarily on the rules and procedures, the student must often resort to gamesmanship to protect himself from aversive control measures. Affective learning is then directed toward behaviors which are not conducive to accountable professional practice.

Alfred Kadushin discusses this issue in his article, "Games People Play in Supervision." Recognizing that games are played because of the payoff received, he states, "One party to the games chooses a strategy to maximize his payoff and minimize his penalties. He wants to win rather than to lose, and he wants to win as much as he can at the lowest cost."[4]

Evaluation: Theory and Strategies

Do some of the following games sound familiar to you?

1. **Be Nice to Me Because I Am Nice to You** — Play is seduction by flattery. "You're the best clinical instructor I ever had." "You're so helpful." It is a game of emotional blackmail.

2. **Protect the Sick and Infirm or Treat Me, Don't Beat Me** — Learner asks help in solving personal problems. Demand now is therapist-client, rather than teacher-learner. Now a payoff is in softer demands.

3. **Evaluation is Not For Friends** — Redefines the relationship to a social relationship and thereby vitiates the professional component of the relationship.

4. **If You Knew Dostoyevsky Like I Know Dostoyevsky** — Establishes power of knowledge disparity and reverse teacher-student relationship.

5. **Heading Them Off at The Pass** — Learner knows he is doing poorly so he starts conference by freely admitting his mistakes. Since self-derogation is going on, the faculty can only respond sympathetically.

These are only a few of the games that Kadushin mentions, but I am sure they are familiar to you. With this activity as the predominating pattern, evaluation then relates to skills in gamesmanship, not to competency in attaining the objectives.

Game playing is particularly destructive to affective learning. Some individuals feel that competitive skills and strategies for beating the system are appropriate concerns for educational programs in order to prepare students for the real world. Etzioni challenges this concept for he sees the role of the school to educate individuals morally beyond prevailing society standards so that they have some ethical principles with which to make the necessary choices and compromises.*

But need gamesmanship be the predominating pattern? It must be remembered that games can be played only when the teacher also agrees to enter into the activity. The controller is most liable to be the participant in game playing, for often it is the outcome of the learning, not the process itself, that is the focus of evaluation. With this emphasis, the means of learning become less significant to the learner.

What of evaluators who perceive of evaluation for growth? These individuals accept the concept that most learners have the potential for mastery of the learning tasks and use evaluation as a diagnostic process by which teaching strategies are prescribed to stimulate the learner's search

*Etzioni A: Do as I say, not as I do. New York Times Magazine, 26 September 1976, p 66.

Dorothy Reilly

for knowledge, values, and practice competency. The climate for evaluation is supportive, based on trust and respect for the learner. The process of development as well as the end result is the concern of these evaluators. Games are minimized, for the teaching-learning process is a shared enterprise. Evaluation is an integral part of the total educational process.

The teacher's beliefs about the nature of man and the teaching-learning process are directly related to his beliefs about the evaluation process and the nature of evaluation strategies developed.

A behavioristic approach to teaching uses evaluation as a means of control. The expected outcomes are specifically delineated as well as the conditions of learning and the criteria used to determine achievement. It is an outcome evaluation approach. All learners and teachers are asked to follow the "same drummer." Although aversive techniques for failure to achieve are not considered a part of this theory, they are indeed used. In many instances the withholding of the reward may be considered aversive. I wonder how often we use this approach with nursing students in the clinical setting when we allow students to have certain experiences only when competency has already been demonstrated rather than looking at the experience as a part of the learning process. I might suggest here that you keep track of how frequently you use the words, *allow* or *let,* in your discussion about student's experiences. The concept of permission to learn is an interesting one.

A humanistic approach uses evaluation as an assessment for growth. It is a dynamic open-ended process closely interwoven with the teaching-learning process. It emphasizes process as well as outcomes. Evaluation for growth is a means, not an end; it enhances the learner's personal development.

An evaluation protocol which is geared toward growth of the learner includes both summative and formative evaluation. Summative evaluation occurs at the end of a program, course, or unit, and refers to the extent to which the learner has realized the objectives which have been specified. This is the most common form of evaluation practice and is used as a basis for deciding grades. Tests, papers, and projects are the usual procedures. This evaluation is addressed to *what is.*

Formative evaluation, on the other hand, occurs throughout the program course or unit and refers to learner's progress toward realization of the behavioral objectives. This type of evaluation is operant throughout the learning process and says *what is* and *what can be.* It relies on the principle of feedback to guide the learner and teacher to those aspects of the learning which need critical attention as the learner moves toward mastery of the behavior. Procedures used include anecdotal notes, problem solving situations, nursing recordings, practice behavior observations, conferences, and videotaping.

This type of evaluation is not designed for data gathering as a basis for the grading process. It is used to assess student progress, to diagnose learning needs so that remedial measures can be instituted promptly, and to pace the student's learning according to his own needs and abilities.

A systematic approach to the evaluation of affective learning, incorporating summative and formative evaluation processes, is required. Objectives expressed in behavioral terms are stated as outcomes consistent with the level of learning expected. Data to be collected and strategies to be developed are determined by these behaviors. Summative evaluation can be achieved and formative evaluation recognizes the developmental aspect of affective learning.

Taxonomy of Affective Evaluation

The objective of evaluation of affective learning relates to two aspects: the experiencing behaviors of the learner which may be evidenced verbally or nonverbally, and the critical thinking process behaviors so vital to the element of choice in value development.

Experiencing behaviors relate to student performance. Krathwohl et al differentiate between *can do* behavior characteristics of the cognitive domain and the *does do* behavior of the affective domain. Recognizing that schools reward students who can do, they say, "In many instances producing the 'right' answer is not so much a matter of ability or previous learning. It is more a matter of perceiving that a behavior which is already in the student's repertoire is appropriate and expected at a given time."[5] Data on does do behavior need to be collected over a period of time and from varied evaluation strategies to evidence a pattern of behavior.

The "Taxonomy of Affective Evaluation" is an illustration of how a professional standard of nursing practice may be appraised in a nursing program. The behavioral objective is stated and then behaviors with appropriate evaluation strategies are suggested for each level of the taxonomy. The listings are by no means complete, and I am sure that the inventive minds represented here could contribute many more ideas. The

FIGURE 5-1†

Taxonomy of Affective Evaluation

I. **American Nurses' Association Nursing Practice Standard**

The client/patient and family are provided with the information needed to make decisions and choices about:

1. Promoting, maintaining, and restoring health
2. Seeking and utilizing appropriate health care personnel
3. Maintaining and using health care resources

II. **Behavioral Objective**

The student provides necessary information to patients/clients and families which will enable them to make decisions and choices on matters related to their own health care.

III. **Behaviors and Evaluation**

Behaviors	*Evaluation Strategies*
A. Receiving 1. Shares ideas with colleagues about nurses as information givers 2. Reports on observation of nurses as information givers	1. Group discussion 2. Written report of nurse-patient interactions
B. Responding 1. Responds to suggestion that he/she provide information to client 2. Expresses satisfaction in instructing client 3. Seeks opportunities to provide clients with information	1. Anecdotal notes 2. Written reports of interaction 3. Clinical conference reporting 4. Log of clinical activities
C. Valuing 1. Takes responsibility for informing client 2. Meets information needs of client in a consistent pattern 3. Supports her/his information activities in a rational manner	1. Series of anecdotal notes 2. Process recording 3. Log of clinical activities 4. Videotaping 5. Care plans 6. Nursing care recording

Evaluation: Theory and Strategies

D. **Organization of Values**

1. Is consistent in providing clients with information
2. Formulates a position for the nurse's responsibility to keep clients informed
3. Defends position on nurse as advocate for needs of clients for information

1. Series of anecdotal records
2. Log of clinical activities
3. Videotape
4. Care plan
5. Nursing care reporting
6. Position paper
7. Debate
8. Critical incident reports on advocacy role
9. Seminar presentations

E. **Characterization By a Value or Value Complex**

1. Is accountable for meeting client information needs
2. Serves as a resource to other nursing personnel in meeting information needs of client
3. Evaluates care of other nursing personnel in regard to information giving role
4. Studies client information activities of nurses and other health care personnel

1. Observation reports of practice
2. Written reports of nursing care
3. Critique of care given by other personnel
4. Team conference
5. Studies, research reports

†*Developed from Reilly DE:* Behavioral Objectives In Nursing: Evaluation of Learner Attainment. *New York, Appleton-Century-Crofts, 1975.*

Dorothy Reilly

intent is to suggest an approach to making affective behaviors more precise and to demonstrate the wide variety of evaluation tools we have at our disposal. You will also note that the methods are not new. You are being asked to increase the evaluation dimension of many methods you already use.

The criterion measures for affective learning evaluation are determined from the designated level and need to be concerned with (1) the experience which relates to pattern and affective manner of carrying out the responsibility and (2) the critical thinking process by which the student arrives at the choice to accept this activity as a responsibility of nursing. Cognitive evaluation is also indicated here. Again, it too is determined by the level, for one must have regard for the quality of the information provided in relation to its accuracy, completeness, and appropriateness for the situation and client. This objective is an illustration of the theme throughout this workshop, that cognitive and affective learning occur within the same experience and both need to be evaluated.

Evaluation Strategies

In addition to the evaluation strategies suggested on the "Taxonomy of Affective Evaluation," there are other means of gathering data about the student's affective learning. We are all aware of the importance of communication as a source of data about an individual's motivations. The *how* of the carrying out of nursing actions tell much of what affective component is operating. In the example of the information giving behavior, criteria must consider how that information is communicated. A straight telling process may provide information, but it does not recognize the right of the client to understand the information nor to relate the information to other concerns he might have. One student shared with her classmates that she disliked a particular ethnic group of people and had no use for girls who became pregnant out of wedlock. She reported that her patient was a sixteen-year-old, out-of-wedlock mother of that ethnic persuasion, so she just taught her the bare facts; "what she was supposed to know." Fortunately, the student was able to share her feelings, and the group became directed toward the exploration of alternatives and consequences. How much prejudiced practice is occurring in an out-of-awareness state on the part of the practitioner and

Evaluation: Theory and Strategies

those individuals responsible for the quality of care in a health care setting?

There are other ways that individuals communicate feelings, attitudes, and beliefs. One of the most common is through the use of labels applied to individuals or groups. Do such terms as *culturally deprived, uncooperative, complaining,* or *crock* sound familiar to you? Daniel Dodson, a professor at New York University, referred to this labeling as "infant damnation." A label excuses the individual from helping the person so labeled because nothing can be done. It also excuses the one labeled from having to reach a solution to the problem.

What are the labels that nurses use to categorize clients? A teacher interested in affective learning becomes very sensitive to labeling terms used by students and challenges them to provide support for the use of the label. One group of students with whom I worked carried out a study of patients in a clinical setting who were labeled as uncooperative by the nursing staff. Most were between 60 and 80 years of age, had a terminal illness, and had few visitors. The need behavior exhibited by the patients resulted in their being labeled as uncooperative; their behavior was not understood or accepted by the staff. The staff's behavior of labeling the patients was not reflective of an accepted value of man's inherent worth.

Before leaving this discussion of labels, might I suggest that you record the labels your faculty colleagues use in describing students. One graduate student reported to our class on the labels she heard faculty in her setting use to describe students over a week's period of time. She also noted that some of the labels were ones she used.

Not only are labels significant indicators of the learner's feelings and attitudes, but so are the modifying words used in describing individuals or situations. How often do we use such terms as *all, every, never?* Challenge to defend our generalizations will do much to help us see our tendency to distort an image in our favor. Evidence of sweeping generalizations, identification of phenomena as good or bad, and the use of absolutes in written work or group discussions provide the teacher with opportunity to assist the student in clarifying his/her value stance on issues.

Since values penetrate our lives, data on student's interests and activities are also important in formative evaluations as we help the student develop his/her own value systems. Explorations of the meanings of these activities in terms of either value indicators, or values and their relationship to nursing practice and the professional expectations, will assist the student in the choosing process of value development.

Dorothy Reilly

Problem solving activities provide very good evaluative data on the critical thinking process in the development of values. The complexity of the problem is determined by the level of affective taxonomy, but the problem must require the choice factor on a value related issue. The source of the problems are best selected from the student's clinical practice experiences, the world of the student, societal issues, or hypothetical situations which may be in written form or on some form of multimedia. The problems may be explored in a group setting or may be done in a written form by the student. The focus of the evaluation is on the critical thinking process and relates to the identification of alternatives, the prediction of consequences of each alternative, and the rationale for the first choice. These data provide evidence of the basis upon which choices are made. If questions request that students express a feeling, opinion, or belief, there cannot be a right or wrong response; but the critical defense of the feelings is subject to analysis. If the student's feelings are not compatible with society or professional expectations, then the basis should be evidenced in the critical thinking process, which in itself may be faulty.

The teacher needs to be alert to the possibility that the acknowledged feeling, opinion, or belief of a problem situation may be representative of the expected one rather than the student's true response. After the teachers' intentions are adequately tested and the teachers are accepted as authentic individuals supportive of the students' value search, students will be more honest in expressing their own stance on the issue. However, evidence of the use of the "right response" as a means of protection is in itself a valuable source of formative evaluation data.

Evaluation of the affective domain is possible, and there are many appraisal techniques that you are currently using in your program. I have purposely stayed away from standardized commercial tests on values, interests, etc, for this information is readily available to you from other sources. The intent here is to see the potential that already exists within your programs and to explain ways that these methods can be expanded to place greater emphasis on affective learning.

Many of the suggestions here are appropriate for formative evaluation, and indeed this type of evaluation should be stressed in any nursing program. However, some strategies will also be used to determine the outcome of the value process development. The major concern is that a systematic program for the evaluation of affective learning be instituted that provides for both formative and summative strategies.

Evaluation: Theory and Strategies

Grading of The Affective Domain

Although this paper emphasizes evaluation, I know that questions will be raised as to how the ensuing process, grading, relates to affective learning. I have no supported theoretical position on the issue. However, I do have some ideas that are derived from my own theoretical framework of the educational process.

One criticism is that there are no existing standards for cognitive learning. I can challenge the concept of ready standards for much cognitive learning evaluation. In cognitive learning we are ready to accept the data that show that the student knows (although the validity of the data may even be challenged), but we hesitate to accept or to believe the data we obtain about affective learning.

We do have an ethical code and standards for nursing practice which are value related. We can accept these standards as reflecting ethical and moral behavior. Philosophers, behavioral scientists, and health care scholars are continuing to search for the definitions of the right behavior expected of professionals serving the health needs of their fellowman. Standards are becoming more explicit.

Thus expected standards of conduct can be specified as objectives, and the student can be expected to achieve them. Remember that evaluation is based not only on the experience or the performance behavior, but also on the choice decision as arrived at by the critical thinking process.

When students are asked for opinions, feelings, beliefs, or points of view on value related issues, the opinion cannot be graded. However, the logic, accuracy, and completeness of the rationale for the opinion can be graded.

Value related patterns of behavior that are specified as objectives can be graded as any other behaviors in the cognitive and psychomotor domains on the basis of criterion measures. It is important to bear in mind that the grading of affective behaviors incorporates data from performance and from the choosing process.

The charge to teach and evaluate the affective domain is not made lightly, for it places heavy demands on faculty. Development of values as operational beliefs requires time, patience, and even some pain.

Krathwohl et al discuss the opening of Pandora's box if we become involved in evaluating the affective domain and are forced to face reality. They respond to those who suggest that the box be kept closed.

Dorothy Reilly

It is in this "box" that the most influential controls are to be found. The affective domain contains forces that determine the nature of an individual's life and ultimately the life of an entire people. To keep the "box" closed is to deny the existence of the powerful motivational forces that shape the life of each of us. To look the other way is to avoid coming to terms with the real.[5]

Is nursing ready to open the box? As we prepare our evaluation protocols for affective learning, let us leave room for the student who occasionally speaks to us, thusly:

I MEANT TO DO MY WORK TODAY

*I meant to do my work today
but a brown bird sang in the apple tree,
and a butterfly flitted across the field,
and all the leaves were calling me.*

*And the wind went sighing over the land
tossing the grasses to and fro
and a rainbow held out its shining hand,
so what could I do but laugh and go?*

Richard LeGallienne

References

1. Vanier J: Tears of Silence. Toronto, Canada, Griffin Press, 1970, p 32.
2. James W: Talks to Teachers. New York, Dover Publications, 1962, p 3.
3. Podeschi RL: William James and education. Educ Forum. January 1976, p 228.
4. Kadushin A: Games People Play in Supervision. Social Work. July 1968, pp 13-23.
5. Krathwohl DR, Bloom BS, Mases B: Taxonomy of Educational Objectives, Handbook II, Affective Domain. New York, David McKay Co Inc, 1964, pp 66, 91.

6

Summation

Presented at Conclusion of Workshop

Ann Zuzich, R.N., M.S.

It is hoped that all of you share with me an enthusiastic response to the experience of the last two days. We have been able to get into each other's minds a little — an always stimulating and rewarding process.

We have spent some time on experiential activity to assist us in clarifying our own personal values, and in some instances, on activity which assisted us in identifying conflicts as our personal values meet the professional values to which we are committed. We have struggled with exercises presenting moral dilemmas involving health research, professional accountability, peer review, and professional and personal responsibility. We have debated different resolutions for these dilemmas. We have experienced both identifying and articulating the rationale to support moral decision making and how to defend the logic and completeness of that rationale. We have practiced the use of some strategies to evaluate critical thinking.

Ann Zuzich enabled us to consider the study of ethics as she explored some ethical frameworks that are basic to an understanding of our moral behavior. In our exercises relating to moral dilemmas, we had the opportunity to identify the ethical framework which guides our decisions.

Dr. Castles stimulated our thinking about the development of professional codes of ethics. She encouraged us to consider the weaknesses as well as the strengths in our professional codes. She suggested that conflict with personal values presented all of us with serious dilemmas for which resolutions must be sought.

Professor Waugh presented us with Kohlberg's Theory of Moral Development and guided us through some exercises in the identification of the stages of moral development guiding moral behavior. We learned that there are techniques for learning to function at higher stages of moral development according to Kohlberg's theory.

Ann Zuzich

Dr. Reilly's papers provided us with the theoretical concepts for the teaching and evaluation of values. She challenged us to extend the parameters of the teaching methods that we use so as to broaden the teaching of values. Recognizing the demands that such teaching makes on faculty, she motivated us to pursue the acquisition of skills in this area by using examples indicating the pleas of the consumer for increased competence in this component of care. She challenged us to use our creative ability to expand the numbers of strategies that might be used in evaluating the affective domain of learning. The affective domain of learning is the emotional learning outcome; it is the feeling tone expressed by such terms as *attitudes, beliefs,* and *values.*

Hopefully, we are at the beginning of a more sensitive consideration of the teaching and evaluation of values in health professions. The need is great. The consumer is pleading for our consideration of the need. We must reach for a deeper understanding of the ethical and moral concepts, and commit ourselves in our teaching to a creative use of ourselves in helping our students in affective learning.

Appendix
I. Moral/Ethical Issue Activities
II. Values Clarification Activities
III. Code for Nurses

Appendix I

MORAL DILEMMA

TOPIC: Quality of Nursing Care

Directions:

1. Read the following situation.
2. Briefly jot down the position or action you, as the nurse involved, would take.
3. Share your position or action with members of your group.
4. Identify the various positions or actions of members of group according to Kohlberg's Stages of Moral Development.

Situation:

You are a staff nurse in the emergency room of a large metropolitan hospital. A 21-year-old male who is a known substance abuser is not oriented to time and place but can state his name. Also, he continues to mumble "No drugs ma — no drugs ma." After a brief assessment, Nurse A takes an unscheduled cigarette break and leaves you to watch over all of the patients. Some 20 minutes later when she returns, you suggest she recheck the patient as he is not as verbal as he was on admission. Some 40 minutes later, you inquire how the patient is doing, and Nurse A states, "He'll keep until the doctor decides what he wants to do with him." Two hours after admission you note the patient is virtually motionless. Nurse A is nowhere around. You assess him yourself. All his vital signs are depressed and he is minimally responsive to stimuli. Nurse A then appears, observes you taking the patient's blood pressure and wants to know why you are checking her patient. You share the results of your assessment with her and she states: "His condition must have suddenly changed, I just checked him." The physician appears at which time Nurse A reports the results of your assessment. The patient is diagnosed to have a cardiovascular accident (CVA). Later, you overhear the physician compliment Nurse A on her excellent assessment of the patient's decreasing level of consciousness.

Appendix

MORAL SITUATION

TOPIC: Interprofessional Accountability

Directions:

1. Read the following situation.

2. Briefly state in writing the position or action you as the nurse involved would take.

3. Share your decision with members of your group providing the rationale for your choice.

4. Identify the various decisions of members according to Kohlberg's Stages of Moral Development.

Situation:

You are a staff nurse in the emergency room of a large metropolitan children's hospital. A one-month-old baby is admitted with a fever of 104 F and is exhibiting grand mal seizures. Dr. Smith, the resident on duty, requests you to prepare and administer 3/4 grain of phenobarbital for the child. You advise him that the dosage is excessive and suggest the appropriate dosage. In a loud voice and with his teeth grinding together, he reminds you that he is the physician and proceeds to prepare and administer the drug himself. Following the administration of the drug, the child's seizures subside, she becomes extremely lethargic, and her respirations become very shallow requiring mechanical ventilation.

MORAL SITUATION

TOPIC: Interprofessional Accountability

Directions:

1. Read the following situation.

2. Briefly state in writing the position or action you as the nurse involved would take.

3. Share your decision with members of your group providing the rationale for your choice.

4. Identify the various decisions of members according to Kohlberg's Stages of Moral Development.

Situation:

On an extremely busy day, Dr. Gordon, a first year medical resident, administers an injection of bicillin to a 26-year-old construction worker treated in the emergency room for tissue trauma to the left arm and hand. The patient is immediately discharged following the injection and told to go home and stay off work until he is assessed during his next visit to the Out-Patient Department. He is escorted home by his work supervisor. Shortly after he arrived home, he goes into anaphylactic shock and dies.

Appendix

His family subsequently sues the hospital for malpractice on the part of the resident, stating the husband/father was allergic to penicillin. As the nurse involved with the situation, you recall preparing the penicillin injection for Dr. Gordon and subsequently noted that he recorded in the medical record that the patient was free of allergies and did not record the administration of the pencillin.

You are approached by the family's lawyer and asked to serve as a witness.

MORAL/ETHICAL ISSUE

TOPIC: Research

Directions:

1. Read the situation below.

2. Decide what S. Smith should do.

3. Share your decision with other members of the group.

4. Identify each of the decisions of the group in relation to Kohlberg's Stages of Moral Development.

Situation:

S. Smith, a registered nurse, has been hired to work in the office of a group medical practice. The obstetrician in the practice is interested in identifying populations of women who should not be taking oral contraceptives. He has an ongoing, longitudinal study which began five years ago, and his early findings suggest that age, parity, and ethnic origin all may be related to increased morbidity and mortality rates in women taking oral contraceptives. S. Smith went to the files in order to become familiar with the early phases of the research and did not find consent forms. When she inquired about this, the obstetrician informed her that he had verbal consent, that all the women were told they were in the study, and that he only accepted into the study those women who wanted to take the pill instead of using some other form of contraceptive technique. When she asked the obstetrician how he explained the possible risks to the subjects, he informed her that the subjects were his patients, and they wanted to take the pill, and he did not wish a further discussion.

MORAL/ETHICAL ISSUE

TOPIC: Nursing Research

Directions:

1. Read the situation below.

2. Write down your decision for action.

3. Share your decision with other members in the group.

Appendix

4. Identify each of the decisions in the group according to Kohlberg's Stages of Moral Development.

Situation:

A graduate student in the College of Nursing is carrying out her thesis research at Smithfield Community Hospital. Smithfield is the only hospital in a 100 mile radius, and the only source of data for the student. Her thesis topic is significant for nursing; she is interested in factors influencing maternal-infant bonding which might fall within the domain of nursing control. She has developed hypotheses predicting that bonding is positively related to the amount of contact and the time of initiation of contact between mother and baby. She is utilizing the premature nursery for data collection. Her research design dictates random assignment of all premature infants admitted to either a control group or an experimental group when they have met design requirements of condition and weight. Mothers in the experimental group are encouraged to make long, frequent visits at any time, and are taught and encouraged to hold and to feed their babies; mothers in the control group following hospital practice are allowed to touch their babies without picking them up, and visiting is restricted to twice daily for 60 minutes.

You are the charge nurse on the afternoon shift, and Ms. Smith comes to you with tears in her eyes and asks why she is not allowed to hold and feed her baby like Ms. Jones does. You are aware that Ms. Smith is 36 years of age and an habitual aborter. She and her husband have tried for many years to have a family, and this is their first viable child. There are no contraindications for the interaction she desires, except that her baby is assigned to the control group. Ms. Smith has signed the consent form, indicating her willingness to participate in the study, and the requirements of the design were explained to her at that time.

How will you respond to her?

_____

Appendix

Appendix II

VALUES CLARIFICATION ACTIVITY

Forced Choice

The following statements are expressions of attitudes or opinions.

____1. Death of another person (ages 65-90) brings as much emotional shock and feelings of personal loss as death of a young infant (one minute to one year).

____2. Death from leukemia of a teenage son of a corporation executive causes the health care worker more grieving than does such a death of a teenage ghetto resident.

Activity Instructions:

1. In the space provided in front of each statement place:
   - (A) if you agree with the statement;
   - (D) if you disagree with the statement;
   - (U) if you are uncertain.
     (Please note there are no right or wrong answers.)

2. After each person has marked the statement, have the members of the table count off 1, 2.

3. All with the number 1 take the first statement and come up with a position and supporting rationale.

4. All with the number 2 take the second statement and come up with a position and supporting rationale.

5. Report from group will be:
   - (a) Position and rationale for each statement.
   - (b) Number of A, D, and U for each statement.

VALUES CLARIFICATION ACTIVITY

Forced Choice

The following statements are expressions of attitudes or opinions.

____1. Suicide is more tragic when it occurs among younger people (ages 13-23) than when it occurs in individuals 65 or older.

____2. Death of a community leader by violence is more tragic than such a death of a clerk in a neighborhood store.

Appendix

Activity Instructions:

1. In the space provided in front of each statement place:
   - (A) if you agree with the statement;
   - (D) if you disagree with the statement;
   - (U) if you are uncertain.

      (Please note there are no right or wrong answers.)

2. After each person has marked the statement, have the members of the table count off 1, 2.

3. All with number 1 take the first statement and come up with a position and supporting rationale.

4. All with number 2 take the second statement and come up with a position and supporting rationale.

5. Report from group will be:
   - (a) Position and rationale for each statement.
   - (b) Number of A, D, and U for each statement.

VALUES CLARIFICATION

CONTINUUM

Situation:

Susie is a student in the second year of the nursing program in which clinical practice is provided. The patient for whose care she is responsible has been ordered to have vital signs recorded every 15 minutes because of a potential for physiological instability.

Susie became involved with other activities and forgot to take readings at 10:00 AM and 10:15 AM. She wrote the 10:30 AM readings and then wrote in numbers in spaces for recording the 10:00 AM and 10:15 AM readings.

During a conference later in the day relative to Susie's practice of the day, you noted the recordings she made of the vital signs. You realized that she could not have taken the 10:00 AM and 10:15 AM recordings because both of you were involved in another activity during that period of time.

When you questioned the readings, Susie assured you that she did indeed take the vital sign readings at the designated times. Probing the issue further, Susie finally admitted that she faked the recordings. Two extreme positions are:

1. Pursue the issue no further since no harm was done to the patient.

2. Recommend that Susie be dismissed from the school since she cheated on her recording of patient care.

Task of the group:

1. List as many other possible positions you might take as an instructor.

2. Place these positions in a continuum line between the two extreme positions.

3. Identify where in the continuum most alternatives might occur.

Appendix

EVALUATING AFFECTIVE LEARNING

TOPIC: Analysis of Written Work

Directions:

1. Complete this assignment in preparation for tomorrow's group activities.

2. View the following situation as though you are a pediatric staff nurse in the local children's hospital.

3. Write a one page evaluation (description and interpretation) of the event as though you were recording it for a ward-conference on this patient.

Situation:

For the past four days, you have been caring for an eighteen-month-old child who is hospitalized for an episode of pneumonia. Treatment activities include croupette, intravenous injections, and parenteral administration of antibiotics. The child cries incessantly and says "Mama." The mother has not yet visited the child. You call the mother, explain the situation to her, and request her to visit. She replies that she does not have time, that the child's hospitalization provided her with the only opportunity to visit and help her aging parents since the child's birth. She requests you to "Kiss Mikey for me!"

VALUES CLARIFICATION

TOPIC: Analysis of Written Work

Instructions:

Write a one page narrative expressing your position in support of, or nonsupport of, the following statement.

Statement:

Patients should be allowed to die without excessive intervention methods to support life.

INSTRUCTIONS FOR CODING PAPERS

I. Coding

(Note: All coding symbols are neutral in themselves)

A. Values

1. Put $V+$ sign over those expressions which indicate something the writer is for.

2. Put $V-$ sign over those expressions which indicate something the writer is against.

Appendix

B. **Critical Thinking**

1. Put *G* sign over statements that are generalizations.

2. Put *U* sign over universal statements of words (such as *all, every, none*).

3. Put *Q* sign by qualifying phrases that take away from absolute (such as *maybe, might, in my opinion, some believe*).

4. Put *A+* sign by expressions attributed to other people or things that are positive (adjectives, adverbs, labels).

5. Put *A–* sign by expressions attributed to other people or things that are negative (adjectives, adverbs, labels).

6. Put *R* over statements you think should be re-examined by the writer.

II. **Process**

1. Code the paper of someone at the table according to the above code.

2. Make two columns — one of *V+* items and one of *V–* items (show what one is for or against).

3. Return paper to writer.

4. Writer read coding and think of what it means.

5. Coder asks questions of writer to clarify thinking.

VALUES CLARIFICATION

Values Statement — Letter to the Editor

In the April 1973 issue of the *American Journal of Nursing,** Joseph Fletcher writes a moral defense of euthanasia. He is referring primarily to active or positive euthanasia, the act of helping a person to die, rather than the passive or negative form of euthanasia, in which life-preserving treatment is withheld. The latter he considers to be already a fact in modern medicine.

He makes his defense upon the understanding that humanness is primarily rational, not physiological; that it is personal function rather than biological function which counts; that being human is more valuable than merely being alive. He suggests that if the well-being of persons is the highest good, then either suicide or euthanasia can be justified in some circumstances. The case for euthanasia depends upon how we understand "benefit of the sick," "harm," and "wrong." If dehumanized and merely biological life is "wrong" and not beneficial, then it is morally wrong to refuse to welcome, or to introduce, death.

An article such as this evokes many responses from readers. Following is a letter which might have been sent.

**Fletcher J: Ethics and euthanasia. Am J Nurs 73:670-675, April 1973.*

Appendix

I work in an intensive care unit, and the points that Dr. Fletcher has made in his article are matters of more than philosophical discussion for me, since many times I care for patients who are in coma and remain alive only because of our machinery. I certainly believe that everybody has a right to a peaceful death, and everybody has a right to know when he is dying. However, I do not see how you can say that the only humans are those who are rational. Either a person is a member of the human species or not, and being nonrational does not change his genes any. You cannot ever stop being human. Are mentally retarded persons not human? Are schizophrenic persons not human? Do you lose your humanism when you go to sleep at night, or if you drink too much? Or if you are hurt in an accident, or have a brain tumor and become disoriented and/or comatose? I do not think you can assign people to the ranks of subhuman just because they do not think as clearly as some of the rest of us. I might not want to keep everybody on a total life support system forever, but it is not ethical to deliberately end somebody's life just because he is not competent, and that is what Dr. Fletcher's disciples would have us do.

A. Identify the position taken by the letter writer.

B. What argument does the writer offer to support her position?

C. Do you support the position of the letter writer?

     Agree _____   Disagree _____

D. Provide rationale for your position of agreement or disagreement.

Appendix III

CODE FOR NURSES

1. The nurse provides services with respect for human dignity and the uniqueness of the client unrestricted by consideration of social or economic status, personal attributes, or the nature of health problems.

2. The nurse safeguards the client's right to privacy by judiciously protecting information of a confidential nature.

3. The nurse acts to safeguard the client and the public when health care and safety are affected by the incompetent, unethical, or illegal practice of any person.

4. The nurse assumes responsibility and accountability for individual nursing judgments and actions.

5. The nurse maintains competence in nursing.

6. The nurse exercises informed judgment and uses individual competence and qualifications as criteria in seeking consultation, accepting responsibilities, and delegating nursing activities to others.

7. The nurse participates in activities that contribute to the ongoing development of the profession's body of knowledge.

8. The nurse participates in the profession's efforts to implement and improve standards of nursing.

9. The nurse participates in the profession's efforts to establish and maintain conditions of employment conducive to high quality nursing care.

10. The nurse participates in the profession's effort to protect the public from misinformation and misrepresentation and to maintain the integrity of nursing.

11. The nurse collaborates with members of the health professions and other citizens in promoting community and national efforts to meet the health needs of the public.†

---

†*Printed with permission of the American Nurses' Association.* Code for Nurses with Interpretative Statements. *Kansas City, Missouri, 1976.*